Oriflame
BEAUTY
BASICS

Oriflame
BEAUTY BASICS

HAMLYN

The Diagram Group

Editorial   Susan Bosanko, Gill Freeman, Jackie Havers, Denis Kennedy, Gail Lawther, Mary Ling, Ruth Midgley, Caroline Schuck, Susan Sturrock

Studio   Alastair Burnside, Brian Hewson, Richard Hummerstone, Edward Kinsey, Jerry Watkiss

Illustration   Graham Rosewarne

A Diagram Book first created by Diagram Visual Information Limited of 195, Kentish Town Road, London NW5 8SY, England.

First published 1986 by Hamlyn Publishing, A Division of The Hamlyn Publishing Group Ltd., Bridge House, London Road, Twickenham, Middlesex, England. Copyright © Diagram Visual Information Limited 1986

ISBN 0 600 50299 6
Printed in Spain

Lito. A. Romero, S. A. – D. L. TF. 873 – 1986

Oriflame is synonymous with quality in the world of beauty. Their range of skin care products and other cosmetics combines the best of nature with the best of science and is distributed direct to the home by thousands of fully trained Oriflame Beauty Consultants.
Should you wish to know more about Oriflame and its wide range of products please write to:

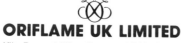

ORIFLAME UK LIMITED

Tilers Road, Kiln Farm, Milton Keynes MK11 3EH (0908) 566531

DSA Members of the DSA

Introduction

Many beauty books seem to assume women have unlimited time and money to spend on themselves. They recommend hours at the gym, days at the health farm and a king's ransom being spent on cosmetics!

But at Oriflame we feel that we know what you really need: informative and practical advice especially for women of today from the Company which produces an acclaimed range of natural based, good-value cosmetics.

Within the world of beauty, the name Oriflame is synonymous with quality. Since its beginning twenty years ago in Scandinavia, the company's reputation for excellent skin care and other cosmetic products has grown and grown. Oriflame employs the most advanced scientific techniques alongside nature's own raw materials – birch, camomile, hawthorn, wheatgerm, witch hazel and many more. All the products are clinically tested on human volunteers in controlled laboratory conditions under the direction of an internationally recognized Professor of Dermatology. This fabulous range is demonstrated and distributed direct to the home by thousands of fully trained Beauty Consultants throughout Europe, America and the Far East.

Now Oriflame brings you a complete head-to-toe beauty book, packed with tips on how to look and feel better. Starting with your self-image and ending with advice on hairstyles, this book takes a fresh and practical look at every aspect of body, skin and hair care.

Chapter 1
well being

Chapter 2
your body

Chapter 3
your face

Chapter 4
your hair

well being

Today's woman wants to look as beautiful as she can within her own physical framework, and to feel at the peak of her health, fitness, and energy all the time. True beauty develops from inside the self, as well as being apparent from the outside. Its essence lies in being who you are and believing in yourself. The basis of confidence and self assurance is a healthy body. Being in shape, at your correct weight, physically fit, and able to cope with everyday stresses and strains will make every sphere of your life that much more enjoyable. Health and nutrition, fitness and exercise, proper relaxation and sleep are just as important for your looks and vitality as a good beauty routine.

Self image

We all have an idea of the way we look, but this image is not always realistic. Sometimes we are too hard on ourselves (seeing only the incipient double chin and ignoring the neat ankles), while at other times we may try self deception (picking clothes that are too small because we refuse to admit we have put on weight). We can all benefit from taking a fresh look at our self image, and by being as realistic about it as possible.

TAKING STOCK: YOUR SHAPE

Start by standing naked in front of a mirror and examining your reflection, both front view and sideways on. Don't pull in your stomach, or clench your buttocks, or try to flatter yourself in other ways. Decide what you really think about your figure and your posture. Look at the tone of your body, at your skin, muscles, hair, and nails. Perform the pinch test (see p. 11), and then weigh yourself.

Make a note of all your findings, and of all the assumptions you have about yourself and your body – the good points as well as the bad. Decide which parts of yourself you can and want to change, which parts you must accept as they are, and which you like and want to emphasise. Distinguish carefully between imperfections you can work on and those you must accept. No amount of dieting and exercise can change your basic inherited body type – but excess weight, bad posture, and lack of fitness have nothing to do with body type!

TAKING STOCK: YOUR LIFESTYLE

Examine the way you feel physically and mentally and the way you live your life, in the same way that you examined your figure. Make a note of all the assumptions you have about what you eat, the way you spend your time, how different activities make you feel, and so on. Then try keeping an accurate, detailed diary for a few weeks. Don't cheat: no one else will see it, so the only person you will be cheating is yourself. Then match your assumptions with the facts. Are you really living the life you want to lead? How may excuses have you been making to yourself – perhaps you really do have time for more exercise? Is your diet really as healthy as you thought? What in your life causes you stress and what can you do about it? Obviously this exercise takes longer than just looking at yourself in a mirror, but you will probably find that the time is well spent. The more information you have, the more accurate you can be in your image of yourself.

SOMATOTYPES

Somatotype means "body type." There are three distinct somatotypes: ectomorphs, mesomorphs, and endomorphs. Although none of us belongs precisely to one of these groups, most of us will recognise our build and body structure as a variation on one of them. It is helpful to know your somatotype so that you can come to terms with your inherited shape: somatotypes cannot be changed.

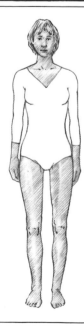

Ectomorph
The long bones and straight, slim shape of the ectomorph are easily identifiable. Ectomorphs are naturally thin, usually long legged, and have very little natural musculature. They may be lacking in energy and vitality. Ectomorphs never seem to put on weight, however much they eat, but may develop poor eating habits, such as a diet containing too much sugar and starch.

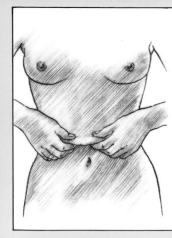

The pinch test
How easy is it for you to pinch a roll of flesh on your upper arm, inside thigh, midriff, or buttocks? Stand upright when you do the test and use your thumb and forefinger to make the pinch. If you can painlessly pinch more than 2.5cm of flesh in these areas, you are overweight.

TAKING CHARGE

Self assessment is the first step in taking charge of your well being. Once you have peeled away the myths and found a realistic self image, you can set yourself definite goals for self improvement. The way you look, the way you feel, and what you ultimately achieve all depend on you.

Make sure that your goals are realistic and worth attaining. Distinguish between the difficult to achieve, which may take time and trouble but which will be worth it, and aiming for the impossible, over which you can have no control. You could perhaps climb the highest mountain – but it is impossible for you to add an inch to your height. Once you have set your goals, start working toward them right away. Stop making excuses and putting things off. Work hard for what you want, try wholeheartedly, and believe that you are going to succeed. Above all, start enjoying everything you are doing. If the changes you bring about make you unhappy, go back to the beginning and rethink it through.

DESIRABLE WEIGHTS

This table gives you a guide to the desirable weight for your height and build. Measuring the circumference of your wrist will give you an indication of your build. If it is 13.9cm or less, you have a small frame; if it is over 13.9cm but less than 16.5cm, you have a medium frame; if it is 16.5cm or over, you have a large frame. Measure your height without shoes and weigh yourself without clothes.

Height	Small frame	Medium frame	Large frame
1.47m	45.4kg	48.4kg	52.9kg
1.50m	46.7kg	49.8kg	54.3kg
1.52m	48.0kg	51.2kg	55.7kg
1.55m	49.4kg	52.5kg	57.0kg
1.58m	50.8kg	54.3kg	58.8kg
1.60m	52.2kg	56.2kg	60.7kg
1.63m	54.0kg	58.0kg	62.5kg
1.65m	55.8kg	59.8kg	64.3kg
1.68m	57.6kg	61.6kg	66.1kg
1.70m	59.4kg	63.4kg	68.0kg
1.73m	61.2kg	65.2kg	70.0kg
1.75m	63.0kg	67.0kg	72.0kg
1.78m	64.8kg	68.9kg	74.3kg
1.80m	66.6kg	71.1kg	76.5kg
1.83m	68.4kg	73.4kg	79.0kg

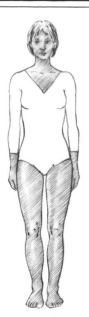

Mesomorph
Mesomorphs may be tall or short, but all are naturally powerful and muscular. Their shape is like an inverted triangle, with slim boyish hips and well developed shoulders. Mesomorphs have a great deal of energy and find exercising easy. They are unlikely to suffer from any real weight problems, provided they remain active.

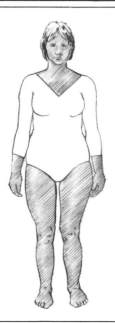

Endomorph
This type is naturally rounded, often plump, and not very tall. Endomorphs have wide hips and heavy bodies, but small and delicate hands and feet. Most endomorphs have a weight problem: they put on weight very easily, and have great difficulty in losing it again. Their body movements tend to be slow and deliberate.

©DIAGRAM

11

Posture

Your posture – how you stand, walk, and sit – can make all the difference to your appearance. If you stand straight, walk tall, and sit comfortably you will both feel good and look good. And if you normally have a tendency to slump, standing and walking tall will make you look inches thinner! Good posture means that you use the minimum amount of effort to balance your body correctly, and so you put the least amount of strain on your muscles. Bad posture is tiring: a person who stands and moves awkwardly wastes a great deal of energy. Once you fall into bad posture habits, your muscles will be pulled and stretched to cope with your body's unnatural movements. This can lead to tension, joint damage, and pain or discomfort.

Be aware of your posture, of how you hold and use your body. Think what you are doing as you stand in a queue, walk along the road, carry heavy bags, or bend down to pick up something from the floor. Remember that your mood can affect your posture, but that in turn your posture can affect your mood. Next time you feel tired and start standing badly, try "pulling yourself together" – improve your posture and see how the tiredness lifts.

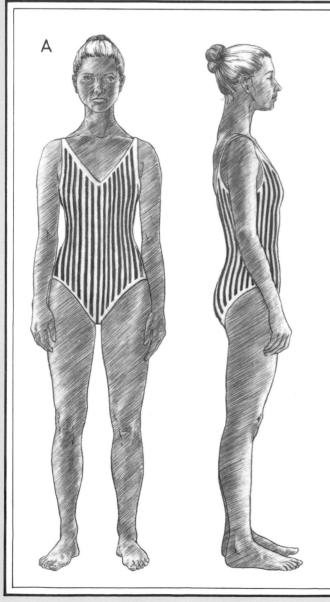

A

CHECKING YOUR POSTURE

Good posture (A)

Good posture means that you are standing straight but relaxed, as if you were suspended by an invisible thread passing through your head, behind your shoulders and hips, and then down through your knees to your feet. If you have good posture, your head will be upright and carried slightly forward; your shoulders will be on an even level, relaxed, and pulled slightly back; and your arms will hang loosely with your hands slightly in front of your thighs. You will keep your chest out and your stomach in, your hips will be on an even level, and your buttock muscles will be relaxed. Your knees will be slightly bent and your weight will be supported on the balls and outer edges of your feet. There will be no sideways curve to your body.

Poor posture (B)

These illustrations show some common posture faults.
a The head is tilted forward instead of being held upright.
b The shoulders are humped and rounded instead of being relaxed and back.
c The shoulder blades protrude, sticking out like wings instead of lying flat.
d The chest is hollowed and the spine curved, instead of the chest being held out and the back straight.
e The pelvis is tilted, instead of being in line with the rest of the body.
f The head is tilted to one side instead of being held upright.
g The shoulders are on different levels, making the back curve sideways instead of being straight.
h The pelvis has a sideways tilt so that the hips are on different levels instead of being even.
i The weight is being carried on one leg and foot, instead of being evenly distributed.

IMPROVING YOUR POSTURE

Because it is difficult to have good posture when your body is in poor condition, almost any form of exercise that strengthens your muscles will help you to improve your posture. Yoga can be very helpful: good, relaxed posture is very important in yoga, and it includes many exercises that are designed to help the spine. Another helpful exercise system is the Alexander technique, which was formulated and developed by Frederick Matthias Alexander, a Tasmanian who spent his working life making an intensive study of the ways in which we hold and use our bodies. When you learn the Alexander technique you are taught how to use all your bones and muscles correctly, especially your spine. Practitioners of the technique believe that it should only be taught on a one-to-one basis or in very small classes, because detailed, skilled analysis of each individual is needed before the correct exercise programme can be prescribed.

POINTS TO WATCH

● When carrying heavy weights, try to balance the load evenly on each side of you. This will help to prevent you developing a sideways curve in your spine.
● When picking objects up from the floor, bend at the knees (instead of from the waist) and keep your back straight. This will help to prevent you developing a rounded spine, and will also put less strain on your back.
● When you sit down, make sure that your pelvis touches the back of the chair and that your back is properly supported. This will help to prevent you developing rounded shoulders.

B

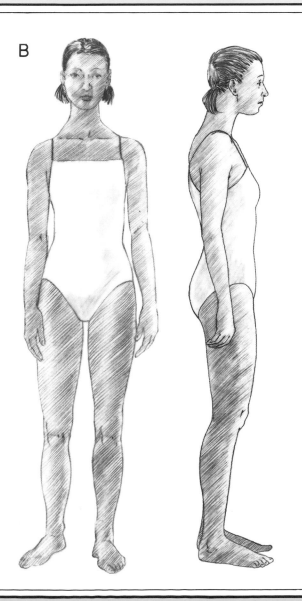

How to check

1 Start by looking at yourself in a full-length mirror, first full face and then sideways. How does your posture compare with illustrations (**A**) and (**B**)? Ask a friend for her comments – she may notice points that you have missed.

2 Next stand two inches away from a wall with your back toward it, feet hip width apart. Sway backward until you touch the wall, and note which parts of your body touched first.

If your bottom and shoulders touched first and at the same time, you are standing correctly.

If one side of your body touched before the other, you are not centrally balanced.

If your bottom touched first, you have a tilted pelvis.

If your shoulders touched first, your back is too rigid and your pelvis is thrust too far forward.

If your back touched first, you are rounding and hunching your shoulders. You may find it worthwhile pinning up a sheet of paper marked into large squares (dressmakers' graph paper would be suitable) before you begin the wall test. Your friend can then mark the position of your shoulders, hips and so on, and you will easily be able to see if they are level. Try this test sideways on as well.

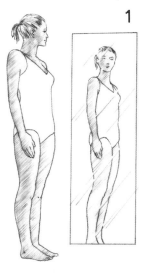

1

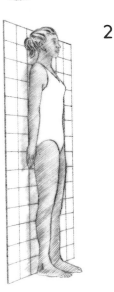

2

Calories defined
Energy provided in the form of food is measured in calories. A calorie is the amount of energy needed to raise the temperature of 1cc of water by 1°C. The measure used for food is 1000 times this, and is sometimes referred to as a kilocalorie (kcal). Most people refer to kcals as calories (cals) as we do here. Another unit used for measuring food energy is the joule. One calorie equals 4.2 joules.

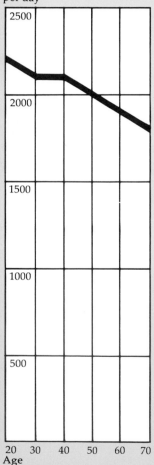

Calories and age
This diagram shows how age affects the daily calorie requirements of a typical woman living in a temperate climate.

Food is essential for all of us. It is the fuel that gives us energy and keeps our bodies functioning efficiently. It is important to know how much as well as what types of food we need to be healthy. The amount of food you need depends on your individual body chemistry, as well as on a variety of other factors: your age, your size, how physically active you are, whether or not you are pregnant, and so on. If you eat more than you need, you will become overweight; if you eat less than you need, you will lose weight.

CALORIES AND AGE
Your calorific requirements will vary with age. Between 18 and 22 you will need 2100 calories a day on average. From 23 to 50 you will need fewer, about 2000 a day, and from 51 onward you will need only about 1800 a day. As people get older they tend to become less active and their metabolism slows down: you will therefore need fewer calories to maintain a steady weight level.

SPECIAL NEEDS
There are certain circumstances in which you will need more calories than usual, e.g. during pregnancy and when breastfeeding. At one time it was thought that when pregnant you should "eat for two": this is no longer thought desirable. In fact, you need to take care not to gain excess weight when pregnant. During the second part of your pregnancy you will need to increase your calorie intake, but only slightly. Opinions vary about the exact size of the increase, but an average of 2250 calories a day in total should be enough. This figure assumes that you will be taking less exercise than usual at this stage in your pregnancy.
If you breastfeed, you may find that you feel hungrier and thirstier than usual. This is because your calorie needs have increased. On average you will need an extra 500 calories per day while you are breastfeeding.

CALORIES AND EXERCISE
Your body is using calories every second of the day, even when you are asleep. You need about 1450 calories just to keep alive. Your exact calorific requirements will vary with your level of activity. If your work is sedentary, you will only use up about 70 calories an hour, but an hour's dancing will use up 325 calories.

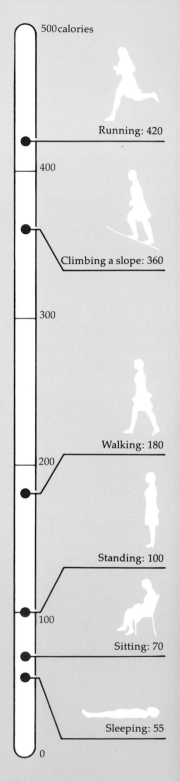

Calories and activity
This diagram compares the number of calories that a typical woman uses up when doing various activities for one hour.

VARIETIES OF FOODS

You can choose the food you eat from a wonderful variety: meat, fish, dairy products, vegetables, fruits, cereals, fats, nuts, seeds, and legumes. All these foods can be grouped into types: proteins, carbohydrates, fats, vitamins, and minerals. These will be discussed in more detail on pp. 16–17. As well as needing food to keep us alive, we also need water, which is found in varying quantities in most foods. Try to eat a balanced diet that does not exceed your own personal calorific requirements. The chart below should give you some guidelines.

It is based on cooked foods; raw foods usually have lower calorific values.

FRESH OR PROCESSED?

It is much healthier to eat fresh foods rather than processed foods. For example, try to eat fresh fruit and vegetables instead of canned or frozen, or make your own soups from fresh ingredients instead of using packets or cans. You will see from the chart below that fresh foods are less calorific: they are also more nutritious.

CALORIFIC VALUES

These lists show the calorific value of different foods. Except for foods that are normally eaten raw (e.g. fruit), values given are for cooked portions.

Meat	Calories
28g bacon, fried	75
71g roast beef	110
57g kidney, fried	130
71g corned beef	150
99g roast turkey, skinned	150
113g roast chicken, skinned	160
170g ham, boiled	210
113g veal fillet, roasted	260
113g pork chops, grilled	290
170g ground beef	300
113g lamb chops, grilled	315
113g pork sausages, grilled	360
170g lamb's liver, fried	396
142g roast lamb	450
113g takeaway hamburger	450
85g salami	450
113g pork pâté	450
113g steak, lean and fat	500+
1 serving beef curry	500+
142g roast pork	500+
198g frankfurters	500+

Fish	Calories
57g oysters	30
28g caviar	80
85g crabmeat	105
113g cod, baked or grilled	108
170g canned mackerel	350
1 serving fried fish in batter	500+

Dairy produce, eggs	
148ml natural yogurt	80
85g cottage cheese	90
1 large egg, boiled or poached	90
1 large egg, fried	135
296ml buttermilk	150
113g ice cream	220
2tbsp double cream	260
444ml milk	300
113g camembert	360
85g cream cheese	390
113g Danish blue	420

Cereals and cereal products	
1 slice wholewheat bread	75
2 plain crackers	75
28g rolled oats	115
57g spaghetti	210
85g meusli	350
142g boiled rice	500

Vegetables	Calories
142g raw mushrooms	10
142g cauliflower	15
170g lettuce	18
170g cabbage	24
142g carrots	25
198g tomatoes	28
283g cucumber	30
57g boiled peas	40
99g boiled potatoes	80
1 corn on the cob	85
57g potato crisps	140
½ avocado pear	235

Fruit	
½ grapefruit	18
170g melon	30
1 peach	35
1 pear	40
1 apple	50
1 medium-sized orange	55
227g raspberries	56
142g cherries	60
227g blackberries	64
1 banana	80

Fats	Calories
28g low-fat spread	105
28g butter	225
28g coconut oil	225
28g margarine	225
28g sunflower oil	250
28g lard	260
28g olive oil	265

Nuts (shelled)	Calories
28g chestnuts	50
28g coconut, fresh	105
28g walnuts	155
28g almonds	170
28g peanuts	170
28g peanut butter	175
28g cashew	180
28g brazil	185

Legumes	
113g kidney beans	100
113g haricot beans	104
113g butter beans	108
113g lentils	112

©DIAGRAM

Food requirements 2

There are five different food groups that you need for health: proteins, carbohydrates, fats, minerals, and vitamins. You also need water, which is found in most foods. It is important to eat a varied diet, regularly including some foods from each group. Exactly how much of each you should eat daily is a contentious question, as the minimum requirements recommended by some experts may be six to eight times as great as those suggested by other experts.

Few foods belong entirely to just one food group. For example, wholewheat bread is 8% protein, 53% carbohydrate, and 39% water. Its main element is carbohydrate, so it is grouped as a carbohydrate.

PROTEINS

Proteins perform a number of functions in the body. They are needed to repair cells in the digestive system, skin, blood, liver, kidneys, heart, and bones, and also in the production of the hormones and enzymes that control all the reactions that take place in the body.

Proteins are made up of chains of amino-acids. There are 20 amino-acids in human protein and they occur in a variety of combinations. The body can synthesise 12 of them, but the remaining eight, the so-called essential amino-acids, have to be obtained from your diet.

Food protein is classified as either complete or incomplete. Complete protein is protein that contains all eight essential amino-acids; incomplete proteins contain only some of them.

CARBOHYDRATES

The principal function of carbohydrates is to supply energy. They play a particularly important role in the healthy functioning of the central nervous system, the internal organs, and the contractions of the heart and muscles.

Carbohydrates are found in all starches, sugars, and cellulose. In the body most starches are broken down into glucose, which is circulated in the bloodstream, providing fuel wherever it is needed. Under some conditions, glucose is converted to glycogen and stored in the liver.

FATS

Fats are essential to the diet. During digestion they are broken down into glycerin and fatty acids. The body can synthesise some fatty acids from other sources, but three essential ones can be made only from fats.

Fats are important in relation to vitamins, since they act as carriers of the fat-soluble vitamins, A, D, E, and K. These cannot be absorbed from the intestines into the blood without fat and bile. Fats stimulate bile production and that of the fat-digesting enzyme, lipase.

There are two different kinds of fats: saturated fats, and unsaturated – often known as polyunsaturated – fats. Saturated fats have been linked with high cholesterol levels and blood disease, and it is thought that eating unsaturated fats is healthier.

VITAMINS

Vitamins are organic compounds that are found in food and are essential to health. They are known as co-enzymes: they work with enzymes to effect chemical changes in the body. There are about 40 known vitamins: some, such as vitamins A, D, E, and K, are fat soluble, while others, such as vitamin C, are water soluble. Of the 40, 12 are essential for health and must be included in your diet. Your body can make one vitamin, vitamin D, from sunlight. A deficiency of any of the 12 essential vitamins may lead to illness.

MINERALS

As well as vitamins, the body needs 20 essential minerals. Minerals are inorganic substances present in food and water. They are needed to regulate body fluids and the balance of chemicals within the body. Mineral deficiencies can cause illness, e.g. too little iron in the diet can cause anaemia. Different minerals are needed by your body in different amounts. You need larger amounts of sodium, potassium, calcium, magnesium, phosphorus, chlorine, and sulphur than you do of iron, zinc, copper, manganese, cobalt, and iodine. Very small amounts (traces) of chromium, nickel, vanadium, tin, molybdenum, selenium, and fluorine are also needed. The level of minerals present in food is related to the type of soil in which it was grown: mineral-rich soil will produce mineral-rich foods.

SODIUM, POTASSIUM, CHLORINE

Sodium, potassium, and chlorine are minerals that work together to balance your body fluids. They are excreted daily in your urine, the amount lost being equal to that eaten. For a healthy body you need equal quantities of sodium and potassium. You eat sodium chloride in the form of table salt, but it is also found in most fresh vegetables and in large quantities in many processed foods. Experts suggest that eating too much salt is unhealthy. Potassium is found in most foods but particularly in vegetables.

Water content
This list gives the average percentage of water in some common foods.

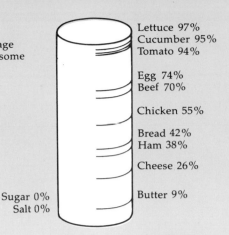

Lettuce 97%
Cucumber 95%
Tomato 94%
Egg 74%
Beef 70%
Chicken 55%
Bread 42%
Ham 38%
Cheese 26%
Butter 9%
Sugar 0%
Salt 0%

Complete animal proteins
Meat, especially liver and kidneys
Fish
Eggs
Milk, whole and skim
Cheese

Incomplete animal proteins
None

Complete plant proteins
Brewer's yeast
Cereal germ
Soybeans

Incomplete plant proteins
Cereals
Legumes: chick peas, kidney beans, lentils, haricot beans
Nuts
Rice
White flour
Wholemeal flour

Condiments
Sugar syrup
Honey
Jams

Cereals and cereal products
White flour
Oatmeal
Chocolate biscuits
White bread
Wholewheat bread

Fruits
Dates, dried
Figs, dried
Peaches, canned
Bananas

Legumes
Baked beans, canned
Haricot beans

Saturated fats
Lard
Butter
Coconut oil
Cocoa butter
Palm oil

Polyunsaturated fats
Corn oil
Soybean oil
Safflower oil
Sunflower oil

Animal foods high in fat
Bacon
Sausages
Pork chops
Lamb chops
Cheddar cheese
Lard or dripping
Margarine
Butter

Plant foods high in fat
Nuts
Cooking oils
Vegetable margarines

Sources of vitamin A
Liver
Fish liver oils
Eggs
Butter
Margarine
Carrots
Spinach

Sources of B group vitamins
Liver   Yeast
Meats   Eggs
Pork   Cheese
Flour   Milk
Bread

Sources of vitamin C
Blackcurrants
Citrus fruits
Green leafy vegetables
Potatoes

Sources of vitamin D
Offal   Dairy products
Fish liver oils

Sources of vitamin E
Vegetable oils
Cereal products
Eggs

Sources of vitamin K
Fish liver oils
Green vegetables

Sources of calcium
Milk
Dairy products
Green vegetables

Sources of copper
Liver   Bread
Kidney   Cereals
Brain
Leafy vegetables

Sources of iodine
Seafood
Kelp

Sources of magnesium
Cereals
Vegetables

Sources of manganese
Unrefined cereals
Wheatgerm
Bran
Green leafy vegetables
Nuts

Sources of zinc
Shellfish
Seafoods
Fish
Meat
Nuts
Whole grains

Healthy eating 1

Although there are many different views on healthy eating, one point on which all experts tend to agree is that you need to eat a varied diet that includes all the different food types. They recommend that you cut down on sugar, refined foods, and animal fats, replacing them with more fresh fruit and vegetables, whole grain cereals, and unsaturated fats.

WHAT DO YOU EAT?

Which of the two menus below most resembles your everyday eating pattern? Menu A is based on processed and fatty foods; Menu B relies more on unrefined and raw foods. Menu B is better for you, as the foods are unprocessed, and either raw or cooked without added fat.

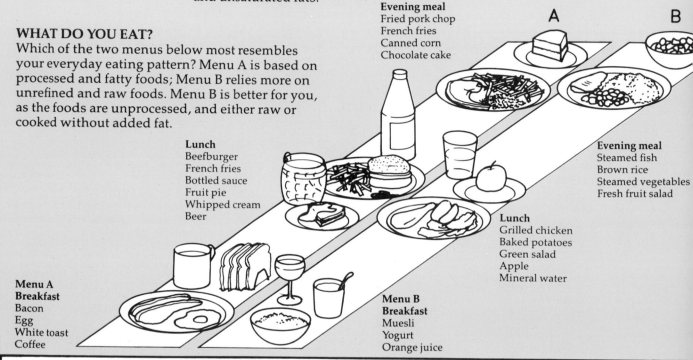

Evening meal
Fried pork chop
French fries
Canned corn
Chocolate cake

A   B

Lunch
Beefburger
French fries
Bottled sauce
Fruit pie
Whipped cream
Beer

Menu A
Breakfast
Bacon
Egg
White toast
Coffee

Evening meal
Steamed fish
Brown rice
Steamed vegetables
Fresh fruit salad

Lunch
Grilled chicken
Baked potatoes
Green salad
Apple
Mineral water

Menu B
Breakfast
Muesli
Yogurt
Orange juice

ASSESSING YOUR EATING HABITS

Do you want to change to a healthier pattern of eating? In order to work out how you will need to change your present eating habits, make yourself a chart using the suggestions below as guidelines. Fill the chart in honestly for two weeks, and see if a pattern emerges. Each time you eat, ask yourself why you are eating: are you hungry, or is it just because it is the time when most people have a meal? Use the information you have collected to help you break your bad habits and plan your new eating pattern.

FREQUENCY OF EATING				
	TIME		TYPE OF FOOD	COOKING METHOD
	STARTED	FINISHED		
Monday BREAKFAST	8·20	8·35	FRESH	RAW
LUNCH	12·05	12·20	CONVENIENCE	BOILED
SUPPER	7·10	7·30	FRESH	STEAMED
Tuesday BREAKFAST	8·15	8·30		
○ LUNCH	12·10	12·25	FRESH	FRIED
			FRESH	STEAMED
Wednesday				
Thursday				
Friday ○				
Saturday				
Sunday				

Frequency of eating
Time started
Time finished
What eaten
List what you have eaten
    every time you eat
What type of food
Convenience
Fresh
Cooking method
List how food was cooked,
    i.e. raw, fried, steamed, etc

Position in which you eat
Sitting
Standing
Walking
Running
Lying
Effects of eating
Repleteness
Hunger
Physical discomfort

BUYING AND PREPARING YOUR FOOD
● Always choose ingredients that look and smell fresh.
● Fruit and vegetables should not be wilted or discoloured. Cracked or wilted vegetable leaves indicate a mineral deficiency in the plant: avoid them as they will not provide you with the necessary minerals.
● Cut down on red meat, eat white meat and fish instead.
● Choose brown rice, wholewheat bread, wholewheat flour, and wholewheat pasta in preference to their white equivalents.
● Whenever possible, eat fruit and vegetables raw.
● If you boil vegetables, a lot of the vitamins will be destroyed. Some of the vitamins will pass into the cooking liquid, so keep it to use as stock.
● Try to eat at least one salad a day.
● Steam fish instead of deep frying.
● Cook foods without adding fat wherever possible, i.e. boil, bake, steam, or grill instead of frying.
● Replace foods high in fat with a low-fat alternative, e.g. use plain yogurt instead of cream.

Know your food
This list shows the calorific changes that occur to 28g of potato when it is cooked by different methods or processed commercially.

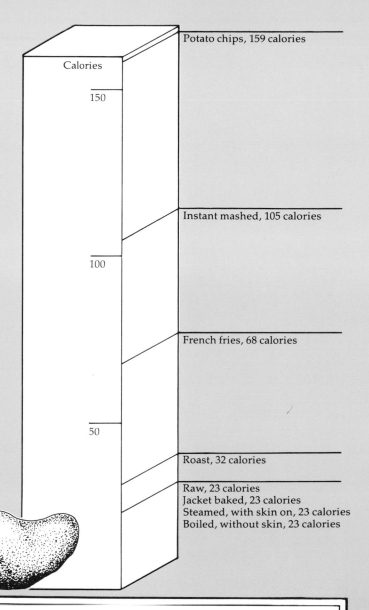

Calories

Potato chips, 159 calories

150

Instant mashed, 105 calories

100

French fries, 68 calories

50

Roast, 32 calories

Raw, 23 calories
Jacket baked, 23 calories
Steamed, with skin on, 23 calories
Boiled, without skin, 23 calories

ALTERNATIVE WAYS OF EATING
There are a number of different healthy ways of eating which may, at first glance, appear a little unconventional. Some people eat only raw foods; others never eat animal produce; still others do not mix carbohydrates and proteins at the same meal. Two of the better known alternative diets are vegetarianism and macrobiotics.

VEGETARIANISM
Vegetarians are people who do not eat meat, fish, or meat or fish products. Some people become vegetarians for humanitarian reasons, because they disapprove of killing animals for food; others simply decide that a vegetarian diet offers them a healthy way of life. A properly planned vegetarian diet is high in fibre and low in saturated fats. There are two types of vegetarian: lacto-ovo-vegetarians, who eat dairy produce and eggs as well as plant products, and vegans, who eat only plants and plant products.
In order to be sure of getting all the essential amino acids they need, vegetarians must plan their meals carefully, mixing incomplete proteins with carbohydrates to give the necessary balance. Vegetarians and vegans include a lot of seeds – sesame, sunflower, pumpkin, etc – in their diet, as these are high in minerals, vitamins, and protein. Vegans may find that a vitamin supplement is necessary, as their diet may be lacking in vitamin B_{12}.

MACROBIOTIC DIETS
Originating in China, macrobiotic diets are based on the ancient Chinese principle of yin and yang. Foods are thought of as either yin (acid) or yang (alkali), and should be eaten in the ratio of five yin to one yang. Foods should also be chosen according to the season and to your state of health. Almost all foods can be eaten, but brown rice is considered to be the ideal food. Some people claim that a macrobiotic diet prevents disease; others have suggested that it may lead to iron and vitamin deficiencies.

Healthy eating 2

In recent years experts have pinpointed four factors in our Western diet that seem to have a direct – and often adverse – effect on our health: too much salt, too much sugar, too much fat (especially saturated fat), and too little dietary fibre.

DIETARY FIBRE

This is the indigestible cellulose found in fruit, vegetables, and unrefined cereals. Fibre is essential in a healthy diet, even though it passes through the gut virtually undigested. The digestive system uses the undigested fibre to remove toxic substances from the body quickly, before they can pass into the bloodstream. Diets high in fibre help to produce soft, bulky, and easily evacuated stools. Cooking vegetables and fruit tends to break down the cellulose in the plant cells, so they are better eaten raw whenever possible. Refining and processing also removes fibre, e.g. wholewheat flour and brown rice have higher fibre contents than their refined white equivalents.

FATS

Cholesterol is a fatty substance that is found in the blood. The body needs some cholesterol, but if the level becomes too high, fatty deposits can form on the walls of arteries, reducing their efficiency. Reducing the amount of fat in your diet will help to reduce the level of cholesterol in your blood. Diets high in fat are also a major cause of overweight: keeping down the fat level will help you keep your weight down. As well as reducing the overall level of fat in your diet, experts recommend replacing saturated fats and foods high in saturated fats with unsaturated fats as far as possible.

SALT

Salt occurs naturally in many foods. It is essential to life, but the daily body requirement is very small – just over one hundredth of an ounce. It is widely thought that too much salt in the diet may be a contributory factor in hypertension, strokes, and coronary disease in general. A great deal of salt is still used in the canning and curing industries, so check the labels on all packets and cans before adding more salt to processed foods. In fact, if you add salt to your cooking you may end up eating 30 times as much salt each day as your body actually needs.

SUGAR

Refined sugars (whether brown or white) and refined sugar products are unnecessary in a healthy diet. The body needs some sugar, but can easily obtain it from foods such as fresh fruit and vegetables. These unrefined sources can be used by the body to greater benefit than refined sugars, because they also contain vitamins, minerals, and dietary fibre. Refined sugars are regarded as one of the principal causes of dental decay and obesity. If you find the thought of a diet that does not include sweet things intolerable, try switching to commercial brands of non-sugar sweeteners for use in drinks and cooking.

ADDITIVES

Whether or not you eat a certain food depends to a large extent on its eye appeal. Many manufacturers use additives – emulsifiers, stabilisers, artificial colourings, flavourings, preservatives, and so on – to give processed foods eye appeal. No one as yet knows the long term effects of these additives on our health, but there is some evidence that links them to allergies, hyperactivity in children, and similar problems. Some countries have banned some additives altogether, although they are still permitted in other parts of the world. No additives are necessary in a healthy diet, so you will not come to any harm by omitting them entirely from your diet.

CAFFEINE

Coffee, tea, cocoa, and certain soft drinks all contain the drug caffeine. It is a stimulant, and in excess can cause restlessness, sleeplessness, and palpitations. It is also a diuretic, i.e. it increases the flow of urine from the kidneys. Some people become emotionally dependent on caffeine. Experts recommend that we limit our caffeine intake and that we drink fewer than five cups of coffee a day (or their equivalent in other caffeine drinks). Try changing to decaffeinated coffee or a cereal-based coffee substitute, or choose from a wide range of herbal teas.

FOODS HIGH IN FIBRE

Cereals and cereal products
Barley flakes
Brown rice
Buckwheat
Muesli
Oats
Rye flakes
Brown semolina
Wheat flakes
Wholewheat flour
Wholewheat bread
Wholewheat pasta

Fruit
All fresh fruit, eaten, wherever possible, unpeeled and raw
Vegetables
All fresh vegetables, eaten, wherever possible, unpeeled and raw
Legumes
Chick peas   Soybeans
Haricot beans
Lentils

FOODS LOW IN FIBRE

Cereals and cereal products
Biscuits
White flour
White bread
White pasta
White rice
White semolina

Other foods
Dairy products
Fish
Meat
Processed foods
Sugar
Molasses

FOODS HIGH IN SATURATED FATS

Coconut oil   Butter
Palm oil   Fried foods
Lard   Potato crisps
Egg yolks   Imitation cream
Beef fat   Hard margarine
Mutton fat   Nuts

UNSATURATED FATS

(Wherever possible use cold-pressed oils.)
Sunflower oil
Corn oil
Olive oil
Soya oil

FOODS HIGH IN CHOLESTEROL

Egg yolk
Whole egg
Liver
Kidney
Butter
Heavy cream
Fish roe

CUTTING DOWN ON SALT

Don't add salt to food when cooking.
Don't have salt on the table.
Avoid foods known to be high in salt.
Switch to low sodium salt substitutes (available from health food stores).
Use herbs and spices to flavor your food instead of salt.

FOODS HIGH IN SALT

Breakfast cereals   Potato crisps
Cake mixes   Processed meats
Canned fish   Salted nuts
Canned fruit   Smoked fish
Cheese   Soft drinks
Margarines   Variety meats
Pickles

REFINED SUGARS AND REFINED SUGAR PRODUCTS

White or brown sugar   Chocolate
Molasses   Canned beans
Maple syrup   Fruit yogurts
Cane syrup   Bottle sauce
Cakes   Most processed foods
Biscuits   Jam
Sweets

NATURAL SOURCES OF UNREFINED SUGAR

Apples, pineapples, and other fresh fruit
Dried fruits
Carrots, parsnips, and other root vegetables
Corn on the cob
Milk

Food-related problems

Recent medical evidence suggests that a great many of the health problems of the Western world may be due to the type of food we eat. Not only do we have an adequate supply of food, but also an enormous choice: we can eat what we like, and as much of it as we want. Unfortunately this does not mean that the foods we select are the most sensible choices as far as our health is concerned. There are a number of diseases and disorders that are now common in countries where a Western-type of diet is eaten, which are almost unknown in the rest of the world. Experts suggest that we can significantly reduce the statistical likelihood of developing these diseases and disorders by switching to a healthier pattern of eating, taking more exercise, giving up smoking, and limiting the amount of alcohol we consume.

FOOD AND ILLNESS
Malnutrition should not be a problem in Western countries, but ignorance of what nutrients the body needs may put some people at risk.

Western illnesses
These diseases and disorders occur to a greater extent among those eating a typical Western diet.

Obesity
Hypertension
Dyspepsia
Cancer
Coronary heart disease
Constipation
Appendicitis
Hemorrhoids (piles)
Varicose veins
Diverticular diseases
Dental caries (decay)
Strokes
Diarrhoea
Ulcers

Diet related symptoms
If you suffer from any of the following, your doctor may suggest that you take a close look at your eating habits, as there may be a connection.

Fatigue
Lack of energy
Hyperactivity
Insomnia
Nightmares
Migraine
Headache
Dental caries (decay)
Spots
Dull hair
Dull skin
Brittle nails
Itches and rashes
Indigestion
Diarrhoea
Constipation
Nausea
Joint and muscle pains

OBESITY
Being overweight is not only currently unfashionable, it can also be a cause of ill health. The risk tables drawn up by major insurance companies suggest that the more overweight you are, the greater your risk of disease and the lower your life expectancy. Clinical obesity is defined as weighing 27% more than the recommended weight for your height if you are a woman, or 20% more if you are a man.

Effects of obesity
These diseases and disorders occur to a greater extent among those who are clinically obese.

Strokes
Hypertension
Heart disease
Poor circulation
Palpitations
Breathlessness
Respiratory diseases
Gallbladder diseases
Cirrhosis of the liver
Infertility
Kidney diseases
Hernias
Arthritis
Varicose veins

SUGAR ADDICTION

The amount of sugar in our diet has increased steadily in recent decades. On average, we each consume about 4oz of sugar a day – some as packet sugar, some in cakes, biscuits, and sweets, and some as "hidden" sugar in a wide variety of processed foods. Recent research suggests that this level of consumption may be the cause of a type of sugar addiction that is thought to affect 40% of Americans. The condition is properly called reactive hypoglycaemia (low blood sugar) but we tend to think of it simply as a "sweet tooth". It is marked by bouts of fatigue, headaches, insomnia, depression, and mood swings, and especially by cravings for sweet things.

These cravings occur because an unbalanced or unsuitable diet allows the level of sugar in our blood to fluctuate wildly. When the blood sugar level is low, we develop cravings for sweet things, and reach for sweets or biscuits to gratify our longings. These easily digestible foods provide an immediate lift in our blood sugar level, providing us with instant energy. Unfortunately this energy "high" does not last long. The blood sugar level soon falls, and we crave sweet things again. This craving/bingeing cycle can be repeated several times in a day.

Because we do not need any refined sugar in our diet, it is possible for us to break out of this addiction cycle. Eating balanced meals at regular intervals during the day helps to keep blood sugar levels more even, avoiding fluctuations. Replacing sugary snacks with dried or fresh fruit also helps. Eliminating sugar from your diet will also help you to keep your weight within recommended levels, and to keep your teeth in better condition.

ALLERGIES

In the past few years food allergies have become a recognised subject for serious study. A whole host of previously inexplicable symptoms, ranging from fatigue to rashes and vomiting, may have a connection with food and our reactions to it. There is no one food that affects everyone in the same way: it depends on your individual body chemistry. Sometimes food allergies are very obvious, as in the case of those people who have an immediate reaction to shellfish, which makes them flushed and nauseous. Other allergies are more subtle, and may take some time to track down.

Before you assume that you are suffering from a food allergy, take a close look at your everyday diet. Perhaps you are feeling less than well because your diet is unbalanced and you are lacking essential nutrients or fibre, or taking in too much salt, sugar, fat, and so on. Change to a low fat, low sugar, low salt, and high fibre diet for a few weeks, and see if the symptoms persist.

If you still suspect that you are suffering from a food allergy try keeping a diary of what you eat, noting down how you feel after each type of food. If your meals include processed foods, remember to read the labels carefully so that you know exactly what you are eating. Your diary may help you to pinpoint the food that is causing the problem. If not, try cutting out one food or food group from your diet at a time (e.g. excluding all dairy products, or all grain products, and so on) until you discover the effect that it has been having on you. In this way you may be able to narrow down and hopefully eliminate the foods that are causing your symptoms. Alternatively, consult your doctor who may be able to refer you to a specialist in food allergies.

Allergic symptoms
Listed here are some of the symptoms reported by patients suffering from food allergies.

Headache
Migraine
Nausea
Dizziness
Vomiting
Depression
Lethargy
Respiratory problems
Rashes
Muscle pains
Hyperactivity
Mood swings

Allergens
The foods, colourings, and flavourings listed here are among those most commonly reported as the causes of food allergies.

Shellfish
Chocolate
Orange juice
Red wine
Whiskey
Eggs
Cow's milk and milk products
Cheese
Coffee
Gluten-containing grains (e.g. wheat, rye, oats)
Monosodium glutamate (msg – a flavour enhancer used in Chinese and processed foods)
Tartrazine (colouring used in orange-flavoured drinks, etc.)

Reducing diets

If you normally eat a healthy diet, i.e. one that is low in fat, salt, and sugar but high in fibre, you are unlikely to have weight problems. However, if for some reason you are unhappy with your weight and figure, you may decide to go on a reducing diet.

There are an ever increasing number of diets and diet foods on the market, some of which are effective, some of which are suspect. As with most things, there are fads and fashions in diets. Think carefully before you choose a diet, and pick one that not only suits your personality and lifestyle but that also offers you a balanced range of nutrients. There is no point in losing weight on a

CALORIE COUNTING

This is a well tried and effective method of losing weight. It is very flexible: booklets giving the calorie counts of all types of food are easily available, so you can plan your own meals. As long as your calorie input is less than your energy output, you will lose weight.

If you work in a sedentary job, and do not take a great deal of exercise, you should be able to lose weight on an intake of 1000 calories a day. If you are very active, you may be able to allow yourself 1500 calories. Choose a calorie count that is realistic for you so that you will be able to sustain your diet easily. A suggested menu for a day on 1000 calories is shown here.

FOOD GROUP DIET

This is a simplified version of a calorie counting diet. Foods are divided into three groups. Foods from the first group are high in calories and should be excluded from your diet. Foods from the second group should be eaten only occasionally and in moderate quantities. Those in the third group are the lowest in calories and can be eaten freely. If you have not lost weight after two weeks on this eating plan, the problem is not what you are eating but how much! Reduce the size of your portions, especially of foods in the second group.

Omit	Eat sparingly
Fatty meats such as bacon, pork, etc	Lean meats such as lamb and beef (remove all visible fat)
Sausages, pâtés, and processed meats	Beans
Duck, goose	Oily fish or fish canned in oil
Butter, margarine, cream, and ice cream	Pasta, rice, cereals, and bread
Cooking oils and fats	Low fat spreads
Thick gravies, sauces, and custards	Eggs
Cookies, cakes, candies, pastries, and puddings	Whole milk and whole milk products (cheese, yogurt, etc)
Dried fruit	
Fruit canned in syrup	
Sugar, jam, honey, syrup, and molasses	

HIGH FIBRE DIET

The average American eats only 113g of dietary fibre a day; on this diet you are recommended to eat twice as much. As well as being good for your general health, high fibre foods are very useful when you are slimming. They take longer to chew and are more satisfying, so you need to eat less of them less often. And because your body converts them into sugars slowly and steadily, you are less likely to suffer from cravings for sweet foods caused by wild fluctuations in your blood sugar levels.

If you decide to follow a high fibre diet, you will need to watch the number of calories you consume as well as the amount of fibre. Books are available

LOW FAT DIET

Fats are the highest calorie foods of all. By reducing the amount of visible and hidden fat in your diet, you automatically reduce the number of calories you are eating. Reducing the amount of fat in your diet is also good for your general health. On this diet you may eat as much as you like of a wide range of fresh fruits and vegetables, providing that they are eaten raw or cooked without fat. The amount of other foods that you eat must be limited to give you a total of between 7 and 10 fat units a day. Books are available which list the fat unit content of various foods, so that you can make up your own choice of menus. Fat equivalent units are also listed for foods which, although they contain little or no fat, contain a large number of calories and little or no nutritional value (e.g. sweets, alcoholic drinks, etc).

diet that leaves you lethargic and with dull hair and skin because you have been missing out on essentials. If you want to lose only a few pounds in weight, you may be tempted to follow a very strict diet or one of the gimmick diets that permit you only a very limited range of foods. These diets might provide you with the incentive you need to lose the weight, but you should not follow them for more than seven days before returning to a more balanced pattern of eating.

The only really effective way to lose weight and to stay at your lower weight is to follow a well-planned diet that lets you lose .91–1.37kg a week, while at the same time getting you into sensible eating habits. If you increase the amount of exercise you take at the same time as you reduce the amount you eat, you will see changes in your figure much more quickly.

SAMPLE MENU
Breakfast
½ grapefruit (with artificial
    sweetener if required)
Boiled egg
1 slice wholewheat toast,
    lightly buttered, with 1tsp
    honey
Total: 255 calories

Lunch
Tuna, lettuce, and tomato
    sandwich on wholewheat
    bread
1 apple
Total: 240 calories

Supper
113g roast chicken, served
    with small jacket potato,
    113g peas, and medium
    piece of broccoli
4tbsp fresh raspberries with
    14.8ml low fat yogurt
Total: 400 calories

Daily allowance of 17.8ml
    milk for drinks: 110
    calories

Eat freely
Chicken or turkey without
    skin
Veal
Vegetables
Fresh fruit, fruit juice, and
    fruit canned in fruit juice
Skim milk and skim milk
    products (cottage cheese,
    yogurt, etc)
Non-oily fish or fish canned
    in brine
Shellfish
Clear soups
Bran
Tea, coffee, water, and low
    calorie canned drinks

SAMPLE MENU
Breakfast
Glass orange juice
Unsweetened cereal with
    skim milk

Lunch
Large mixed salad with
    yogurt dressing

Evening meal
Clear soup
Small portion grilled lamb
    with green vegetables and
    baked potato
Fresh fruit salad

that give selections of fibre-counted and calorie-counted meals from which you can choose your daily menu. In addition you may have as many low calorie drinks as you wish, although fruit juices are forbidden. You are advised to drink a half pint of skim milk and to eat two pieces of fresh fruit daily.

SAMPLE MENU
Breakfast
Wholewheat cereal served
    with extra bran, few
    sultanas, and skim milk
1 orange

Lunch
Spinach and poached egg
    with mushrooms
Watercress salad
1 pear
Evening meal
Chilli beef and beans
Baked apple with banana and
    walnuts

SAMPLE MENU
Breakfast
Orange juice
57g muesli with skim milk
Grilled tomatoes on
    wholewheat toast
Total: 1½ fat units

Lunch
170g grilled chicken (no skin)
Large salad served with oil-
    free dressing
14.8ml low fat yogurt
Total: 2½ fat units

Supper
½ melon, sprinkled with
    ginger
Grilled trout served with
    selection of cooked fresh
    vegetables
42g Brie or Camembert
    cheese, with bunch of
    grapes
Total: 6 fat units

Stress 1

Have you ever felt that you were unable to cope with life, that it was just too much for you? If you have, you were probably suffering from stress. Stress is one of the commonest twentieth century problems, and can affect you at any stage in your life. Pressures and emotional upheavals are part of all our lives, but their mental and physical effects vary from person to person. You need to learn to recognise which situations are most stressful for you, and to find ways of decreasing any adverse reactions.

The biological origin of stress lies in the "fight or flight" response we once needed to stay alive in a world where we had either to overpower our prey or be overpowered by it. Today the pressures are more often psychological rather than life threatening, but our bodies react in the same way to a confrontation with a friend or a colleague as they once would have done to a confrontation with a sabre-tooth tiger. If we let these reactions get out of hand, we risk making ourselves ill: stress can aggravate a wide variety of physical and psychological disorders.

Too little stress can be as bad for you as too much. Some people even thrive on high levels of stress, e.g. competitors who take part in dangerous sports, or people who enjoy high powered careers. Anything exciting, stimulating, and challenging produces some stress. Our bodies do not distinguish between unpleasant and pleasant sources of stress. It is important to strike a balance: too much stress may make you ill, but too little will leave you depressed, lethargic, and feeling like a cabbage.

PHYSICAL EFFECTS OF STRESS

Major changes take place in your body whenever you enter into a stressful situation. The pituitary gland in the brain releases the hormone ACTH into the bloodstream. This in turn activates the adrenal glands, which release cortisones and two more hormones (epinephrine and norepinephrine). These substances adjust your bodily functions to deal with the stress. The heart beats faster – sometimes the pulse increases dramatically from about 70 beats a minute to 120 or more. This means that the blood moves around the body more quickly, taking more oxygen to the muscles. The spleen contracts, releasing more red cells into the blood to carry more oxygen. The blood vessels in the skin and stomach constrict, diverting more blood to the brain and muscles. Breathing becomes faster to bring even more oxygen into the body. Supplies of sugar and fat are released into the blood from the body's stores. There is an increase in the substances that help to clot the blood and repair the body tissues. The skin begins sweating, ready to deal with the excess heat produced by the body's exertion. The body is prepared to fight or to run, depending on the source of stress.

Body parts affected
These are the parts of the body affected by stress. If stress continues over a long period of time you may fall ill.

1 Brain
2 Pituitary gland
3 Adrenal glands
4 Heart
5 Muscles
6 Blood vessels
7 Lungs
8 Stomach
9 Liver
10 Spleen
11 Blood system

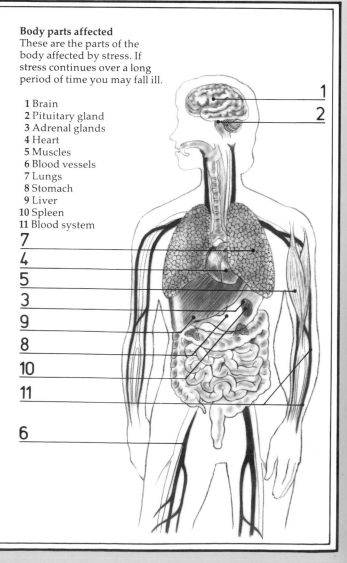

WARNING SIGNS

The warning signs that tell you that are suffering from too much stress may be physical or psychological.

Physical warning signs

If you suffer frequently from any of these symptoms without any physical cause, you may have a stress problem.

Obesity
High blood pressure
Loss of appetite
Food cravings
Diarrhoea
Constipation
Insomnia
Fatigue
Headaches

Muscle spasms
Nausea
Fainting attacks
Inability to cry
Bursting into tears
Hyperactivity
Breathlessness
Impotence
Frigidity

Psychological warning signs

If you suffer on a long term basis from any of these feelings, you may have a stress problem.

Boredom
Lethargy
Uneasiness
Inability to cope
Irritability
Overanxiety about money
Fear of disease or death
Suppressed anger
Rejection

Despair
Phobias
Lack of concentration
Inability to communicate
Personality changes
Humourlessness

EFFECTS OF STRESS

Excessive stress may contribute to a variety of physical and psychological disorders, and can also aggravate pre-existing conditions.

Possible physical effects
Headaches
Exhaustion
Sweating
Hot flushes
Catarrh
Asthma
High blood pressure
Heart disease
Heart attacks
Skin disorders
Indigestion
Ulcers
Aches and pains
Diarrhoea

Possible psychological effects
Depression
Aggression
Alcohol dependence
Drug dependence
Phobias
Hysteria
Obsessions
Anxiety attacks

Body parts affected
These are the parts of the body affected by long-term stress.

1 Brain
2 Head
3 Skin
4 Hair
5 Back
6 Heart
7 Stomach
8 Intestines
9 Pancreas

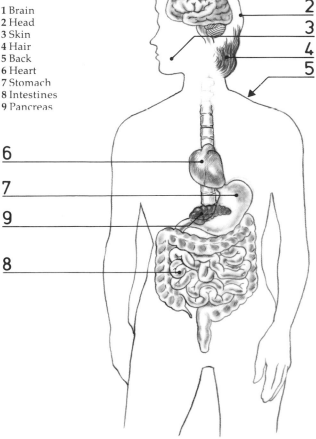

Stress 2

LIFE CHANGES

All the major changes in our lives produce stress. It is easy to recognise the unpleasant sources of stress, but we tend to forget that pleasant events can also be stressful. We need to take them all into account when we are looking at the total amount of stress in our lives. A high stress level can increase our chances of becoming ill or having an accident.

The lists below show some of the major changes in life that can cause stress, and gives each a points score. How many of these changes have occurred in your life during the last six months? If your total score is less than 50 points, you have little stress in your life. If your score is between 50 and 100, the amount of stress in your life is becoming significant: you are 35% more likely to become ill or have an accident than if you were less stressed. These odds increase as the stress level increases – to 50% more if your score is between 100 and 150, and to 80% more if your score is over 150. The higher your score, the more care you need to take of yourself, and you should try to lead as unstressed a life as possible until your score is reduced.

50 POINTS

Giving up alcohol (if dependent)
Giving up hard drugs (if addicted)
Serious personal injury
Major illness
Marriage or remarriage

Divorce or marital separation
Death of partner
Death of close family member
Imprisonment

40 POINTS

Giving up smoking (if smoked over 40 a day)
Major accident (e.g. car crash, fire, etc)
Sexual difficulties
Reconciliation with estranged partner
Pregnancy
Death of close friend

Major anxiety at work (e.g. company failure, strike, etc)
Retirement, redundancy, or dismissal from work
Member of immediate family has major accident or illness or recovers from one

30 POINTS

Enforced unwanted separation from partner
Major arguments with partner
Being unfaithful to your partner
Discovering your partner's infidelity
Gaining a new member in your

immediate family by birth or marriage
Changing your job
Changes in your job (e.g. new boss, new offices, etc)
Major changes in your financial state (for better or worse)

20 POINTS

Achieving something outstanding and receiving recognition for it
Giving up smoking (if smoked less than 40 a day)
Moving house
Major arguments with members of close family

Child starting school, leaving home, or marrying
Starting work for first time
Returning to work after long absence
Promotion or demotion at work
Taking on a debt of more than one year's salary (e.g. mortgage)

10 POINTS

Changes in your daily routine (e.g. the way you travel to work)
Changes in amount or type of your social activities
Changes that affect your leisure interests (e.g. taking up a new sport)
Changes in your sleeping or eating habits (e.g. dieting)

Holidays and vacations
Christmas
Changes in your family or domestic routine
Difficulties with your boss or other superiors
Applying for a large mortgage or loan

ARE YOU PRONE TO STRESS?

You have probably noticed that in a stressful situation, some people cope better than others. Some experts divide people into two groups: those prone to stress and stress-related illnesses are known as type A, while those who are less affected by stress are known as type B. Type A people often create their own stress by their lack of self-confidence. Characteristics relating to both types are listed here; most people are a mixture of the two.

Type A
Competitive
Ambitious
Always in a hurry
Easily frustrated by others
Needs challenge
Always busy
Unable to accept criticism
Unable to express emotions
Eats compulsively
Very gregarious
Workaholic

Type B
Patient
Unhurried
Unflappable
Tolerant
Unselfish
Flexible
Eats only when hungry
Enjoys hobbies
Happy with a few good friends

STRESS AND ENVIRONMENT

How and where you live, work, and travel can make a noticeable difference to the amount of stress in your life. Environment is very important: you will probably have noticed that some surroundings make you feel happy and relaxed, while others make you feel anxious or depressed. The continual noise, congestion, traffic, and pollution of an urban environment are considered one of today's major sources of stress. At the other end of the scale, some people find the quiet and solitude of living in a remote rural area highly stressful.

Try as far as possible to adjust your environment to suit you, so that the stress level is reduced. There is little that you can do about the amount of traffic in the streets or the number of people travelling on your train, but you may be able to alter your route to one that is less popular, or to change your travelling time to a less crowded period. Make sure that the lighting and ventilation at work or at home are suitable for whatever you are doing. Stuffy, smoke-laden atmospheres are uncomfortable, and lighting that is too bright, too dim, or flickering can lead to eye strain and headaches. The colour of your surroundings can also influence your mood, e.g. green has a calming effect, while orange is stimulating. Removing a source of stressful noise can be more difficult, as any degree of soundproofing can be expensive. Earplugs offer a possible solution, or you could try playing your own choice of music through the headphones of a personal stereo.

DEALING WITH STRESS

Each of us finds our own way of coping with the level and type of stress in our lives, but the following suggestions are good points for all of us to remember.

Try to make sure that you are in good physical health. If you eat a balanced and nutritious diet and get enough exercise and sleep, you will be in a better position to cope with stressful situations when they arise.

Try to get a stressful situation into its true perspective. This probably applies much more to everyday stresses and aggravations than to major life crises, which by their very nature are overwhelming. Ask yourself if you are overreacting in stressful situations such as traffic jams, minor family rows, working to deadlines, etc.

Try to talk about your problems with your family and friends, as this can reduce the mental stress that is associated with trying to cope alone. Some problems may be made easier by talking to and taking professional advice from your lawyer, accountant, banker, etc.

Try to make time for yourself. Make sure that you allow yourself the opportunity to take a break from your job or your family to do something different that you enjoy. Strike a balance between work and recreation. Try too to make time to relax (see pp. 32–35).

If the level of stress in your life becomes so high that you are unable to deal with it yourself, seek help. Your doctor may be able to help you, or you may find that individual or group psychotherapy offers a solution.

Cigarettes, drugs, drink

Many people try to find a solution to living with stress by smoking, drinking too much, or using some variety of drug. In the long run, none of these props really helps to lessen the symptoms of stress or to increase your ability to stand up to it. In fact, they can create extra stress in your life if you become dependent on them.

SMOKING

By now we all know that smoking is bad for us, and that if we continue to smoke we are risking serious damage to our health. Smoking is also increasingly regarded as unattractive and antisocial. Many people are now deciding that the benefits of being a non-smoker far outweigh any difficulties they may encounter in giving up. And if you are really unable to give up completely, there are still ways of reducing the amounts of tar and nicotine that you take into your body and so, hopefully, of reducing some of the risks.

GIVING UP

Analyse your smoking habits
Spend a few weeks keeping a record of every cigarette you smoke. Don't let yourself light up automatically. Work out why and when you need to smoke.

Prepare yourself
Really decide that you want to stop smoking. Think about all the benefits that not smoking will bring.

Set the day
Decide exactly on which day you are going to stop smoking. On the night before, smoke your last cigarette, clean out all the ashtrays and put them away, and dispose of any remaining cigarettes, lighters, matches, etc. Then stop smoking.

Change your habits
Your smoking record will tell you when you are tempted to smoke. Change your daily routine to keep away from these trigger situations, e.g. go for a walk after lunch instead of having a cup of coffee. You may find that it will help to give up smoking at a time when your routine will be different from usual, e.g. as you begin your vacation.

Find a substitute
Instead of putting a cigarette in your mouth, chew gum or the end of your pen. If you need something in your fingers, play with a pen or pencil or use a string of worry beads. If you feel the need to inhale something, take several deep, slow breaths of fresh air. If you are tense, practice some relaxation exercises.

Spoil yourself
Save the money that you spent on cigarettes and use it to give yourself a positive reward by buying something you would not otherwise be able to afford. Remind yourself that you were able to afford this luxury because you have stopped smoking.

Be a non smoker
Travel in non smoking compartments, sit in non smoking sections in theatres and restaurants, and so on. Keep as far away from smoking situations as you can. If someone offers you a cigarette, tell them that you are a non smoker.

Give yourself time
Remember that it takes six to eight weeks to break a habit. Don't be tempted back into smoking before you have really given your body a chance to get rid of all the toxins it has accumulated while you have been smoking.

Extra help
If you feel that you cannot give up smoking on your own, there is plenty of help and support available. Nicotine chewing gum may help to relieve any cravings you have; an anti-smoking group or clinic will give you moral support; hypnotism or acupuncture may help to relieve any withdrawal symptoms.

CUTTING DOWN

Change to filter tipped cigarettes with a lower tar content than your present brand.

Even when you are smoking tipped cigarettes, use a cigarette holder that includes a tar filter.

Buy cigarettes that are shorter in length than your normal brand.

Never leave a cigarette in your mouth for more than one puff: put it down in the ashtray after each puff. Try to take fewer puffs per cigarette.

Only smoke a cigarette halfway down its length before stubbing it out, as the last half is where most of the tar collects.

Try to keep away from smoking situations, e.g. by travelling in non smoking compartments.

Do not increase the number of cigarettes you smoke just because you are switching to shorter, lower tar brands. Instead, try smoking one cigarette less this week than you smoked last week.

BENEFITS

These are some of the benefits you can expect if you give up smoking.

Feeling fitter
Fresher breath
Nicotine stains on fingers and teeth will disappear
Improved senses of smell and taste
Clearer skin
Less chance of wrinkles
Clothes and hair will not smell of smoke
Home will smell fresher
More spending money
Improved life expectancy
Less chance of developing lung cancer, heart disease, or other serious illnesses
Less risk to health of friends and family

DRUGS

Drugs are substances that act on your body to change your physical or mental state. Some are available over the counter without a doctor's prescription, some are available only with a doctor's prescription, others are illegal. We tend to associate drug abuse and addiction with illegal drugs such as cocaine and heroin, but legally obtainable drugs can also cause problems. As they have realised the addictive properties of commonly used drugs, doctors have become more cautious in prescribing tranquilizers and amphetamines. It is also possible to become physically dependent on such familiar drugs as laxatives and painkillers.

Once you are drug dependent, it is very difficult to help yourself. You will need to seek professional help from your doctor or a specialised drug unit. It is obviously preferable to avoid becoming drug dependent in the first place. Be sensible in your use of over the counter drugs: you may be able to get similar results without using drugs at all (e.g. if you eat a high fibre diet you are unlikely to need laxatives). Discuss the use of prescription drugs with your doctor, avoid addictive illegal drugs, and remember that alcohol and nicotine are both drugs.

DANGER SIGNS

If you find that you are doing any of the things on this list, you may be at risk of becoming drug dependent and you should seek professional help.

Needing to take drugs to wake you up in the morning and to get you to sleep at night.

Taking painkillers, laxatives, etc, as a "preventive" measure when you have no symptoms.

Taking some form of drug at intervals during the day because you feel you need it.

Keeping drugs in several rooms in the house or always carrying drugs with you.

Mixing drugs to increase their effect.

Taking a drug for its side effects instead of to relieve symptoms.

Being unwilling to admit your exact consumption of drugs.

ALCOHOL

Alcohol in moderation probably does more good than harm, and having one or two drinks is considered a socially acceptable way to relax. Although many of us think of alcohol as a stimulant, it in fact acts as a tranquiliser and depressant. It dulls the brain and nervous system, affecting the parts that control impulsive behaviour, judgment, and memory. We feel stimulated and less inhibited because a drink has temporarily masked our anxieties and fears.

Alcohol becomes a problem when we cease to drink in moderation. Social drinking can become habitual drinking, habitual drinking can become heavy drinking, and heavy drinking can become alcohol abuse almost imperceptibly. Like any other drug taken at the wrong time or in the wrong quantity, alcohol can be dangerous and damaging – for example, it is a major factor in about half of all automobile accidents.

HANDLING ALCOHOL

Drink slowly: the alcohol will then be absorbed into your system less quickly.

Eating before drinking alcohol or eating with your alcoholic drinks will also slow down the rate of absorption.

Dilute your drinks when possible, e.g. add a mixer to neat spirits. It will take you longer to finish each drink and longer for it to be absorbed into your system.

Finish one glass of an alcoholic drink before starting on another: don't just top up your glass.

Don't drink alcohol to quench your thirst.

Don't feel obliged to have an alcoholic drink: have a soft drink if you would prefer it.

Don't drink alcohol when what you really need is rest, sleep, or food.

Don't drink alcohol just to relax: try relaxation exercises instead.

Don't drink and drive.

DANGER SIGNS

If you find that you are doing any of the things on this list, you may be at risk of becoming dependent on alcohol. Ask for help from your doctor or your nearest Alcoholics Anonymous group.

Drinking during the night or first thing in the morning

Drinking alone

Inventing excuses for drinking

Increasing your alcohol consumption

Missing meals or giving up activities in order to drink

Drinking much more quickly than other people

Drinking to reduce feelings of stress, anger, depression, etc

Experiencing severe depression, aggression, blackouts, amnesia, and other behavioural difficulties

© DIAGRAM

Relaxation 1

If you think that you don't have time to relax and that relaxing is a luxury, you're wrong. As life becomes more stressful, it becomes increasingly important to learn to relax your body and mind in order to cope with the stresses. Relaxing plays a very important part in keeping you healthy. As the pressure increases, so your body becomes tense: it needs to be relaxed in order to cope. Try to set aside some time every day for relaxing.

You will need to find out what form of relaxation suits you best. Basically, you need to stop doing whatever it is you do throughout the day and switch to something else: it is the change of gear that is important. Some people find it relaxing to sit and read or sew after a hard day's work. Others like to soak in the bath for a long time, or to go for a swim. Some go to saunas, others have massages. Find time for yourself and do what you want to do at a leisurely pace.

Some of the most beneficial forms of relaxation are physical ones, for in freeing the body of tensions you also free your mind. When you exercise you relax parts of your body that are normally tense, your breathing deepens, and your blood pressure drops. All these things are beneficial to your health.

Try including some physical relaxation in your life. There are a number of approaches you might consider, for example taking up some form of sport by joining a fitness club. You might learn to do breathing exercises or take up yoga – or even just run round the block.

YOGA

Yoga is not only a very useful form of exercise (see pp. 46–47), but also a relaxation technique that involves both your body and your mind. The poses or ansanas help your body to relax, while the breathing and meditation exercises help your mind relax. Most yoga teachers will include instruction on all these aspects of yoga in each teaching session. If you find that hatha yoga (the yoga system most often found in the west) does not appeal to you, investigate one of the many other forms of yoga such as raja yoga or iyengar yoga.

Alternate nostril breathing
This is one of the basic hatha yoga breathing exercises. Sit with your spine erect – either crosslegged on the floor, or upright in a chair. Rest your left hand on your thigh. Put the index finger and the forefinger of your right hand on the bridge of your nose between your eyes. Place your thumb against your right nostril and your ring finger against your left nostril. Use these fingers to squeeze your nostrils together, so closing them. Lift up your thumb and breathe out through your right nostril. Then breathe in through your right nostril. Lower your thumb to close your right nostril and lift your ring finger to release your left nostril. Breathe out and then in through your left nostril. Repeat this sequence several times, making all the breaths slow and deep.

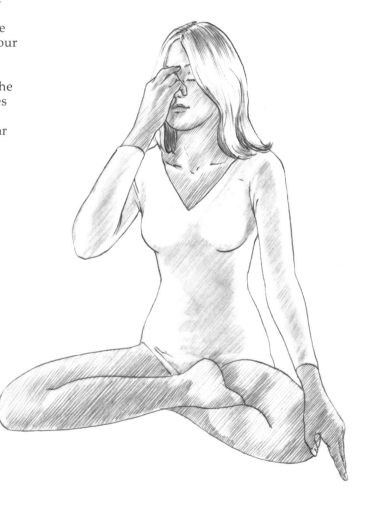

MEDITATION

In recent years meditation has been very much associated with various forms of Eastern mysticism. But there is no need to have a guru in order to use meditation as a very efficient relaxation technique. All you need to do is to learn a meditation technique and allow yourself regular times to practice it – preferably 15 minutes at a time, twice a day.

Research has shown that meditation has many benefits. Your heart rate and breathing rate slow down, your brain waves show a characteristic relaxation pattern, and other useful physiological changes take place. It also has the advantage of making you stop your everyday activities for a time and enjoy a complete change of pace. People who meditate regularly claim that the state of rest that they achieve during meditation stays with them when they return to their usual activities, making them more able to cope with stress and less likely to become anxious, depressed, or aggressive.

When you meditate you focus your attention on an object – a candle flame, or a flower, or even a stone – or on a word (often called a mantra) or a series of sounds which you repeat to yourself inside your head. You keep your attention on this chosen focus. If a distracting thought creeps into your mind, you simply ignore it and return your concentration to your focus. When you are first practising meditation, you will probably find that it helps to sit or lie in a quiet room with dim lighting, and to switch off the telephone and any other possible distractions.

AREAS OF TENSION

Before you can decide which method of relaxation would suit you best, you need to pinpoint the areas of your body that suffer from tension. A good way to do this is mentally to explore how each part of your body feels – whether it aches, feels stiff, is hot or cold, and so on. Find out too whether you register the same sensations on each side of your body – does your right hand feel like your left hand, is your left shoulder stiffer than your right shoulder, and so on.

The easiest way to do this mental tour of your body is to lie down on your back on the floor. Use a pillow to support your head if you wish . Let your arms and legs relax and turn your hands so that your palms are upward. Close your eyes and deepen your breathing. Breathe slowly in through your nose and out through your mouth for about a minute or so. Now start discovering how each part of your body feels. Start with your feet, and then move gradually up your body until you reach the top of your head. If it helps you to get a better sense of a particular part of your body you can move it gently as you think about it. Take your time: it will probably take you about 15 minutes to explore all of you. When you have finished, let yourself relax for a couple of minutes before opening your eyes, turning onto your side, and getting up.

This exercise will have shown you which parts of your body are tense and uncomfortable, and these are the areas you will probably want to concentrate on in your relaxation programme. Ask yourself why a particular part of your body might be painful: do you sit badly, giving yourself back pain, or wear shoes that make it difficult for you to walk comfortably? Removing any causes of physical stress and discomfort will make it much easier for you to relax.

Common areas of tension
Shown right are the areas of the body most often affected by tension. Tension in the back of the neck and the shoulders (a) is usually a result of anxiety. The lower back (b) suffers if you sit badly or otherwise overwork the area. Your leg muscles (c) can be strained by running and exercising.

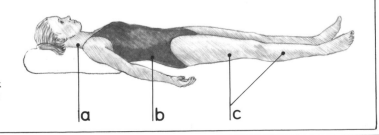

Relaxation 2

In this series of relaxation exercises you work down your body from top to bottom, relaxing each part in turn. Take the exercises slowly and make sure that you don't strain yourself. Get yourself comfortable before you start: make sure the room is warm, wear loose clothing, and get yourself into the right position before attempting any exercises. If you can incorporate these routines into your life you will gradually find that you are more relaxed and less likely to misuse your body. With time your aches and pains will dissolve away and you will feel reinvigorated.

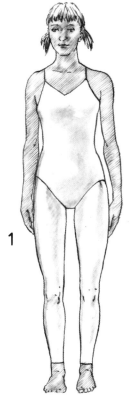

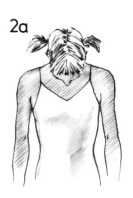

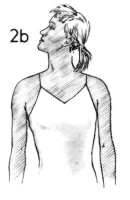

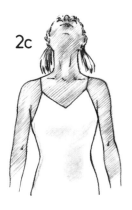

1 Deep breathing
Stand with your feet slightly apart and your weight evenly distributed over both feet. Keep your head up, chin in, and look straight ahead. Let your shoulders drop and your arms hang loosely by your sides. Try not to curve your spine. Now breathe in through your nose. As the air travels down toward your diaphragm, let your ribs rise evenly outward so that there is plenty of space for the air. When you have taken in as much air as you can, breathe it out slowly and steadily through your mouth. Repeat this breathing exercise until you can feel your body beginning to relax.

2 Neck
Stand as for exercise 1. Drop your head forward (**a**), then bring it round to the right (**b**), keeping your shoulders straight. Roll your head back and round (**c**), then complete the circle by bringing it round to your left and letting it fall forward. Repeat in the opposite direction.

3 Shoulders
Stand as for exercise 1. Shrug both shoulders as high as possible (**a**), the drop them as far as possible. Repeat the shrug several times. Then lift your left shoulder as high as you can and swing it back and down, then forwards and up to make a circle (**b**). Still using your left shoulder, repeat the circular movement, but this time begin by moving your shoulder forwards (**c**). Repeat with your right shoulder.

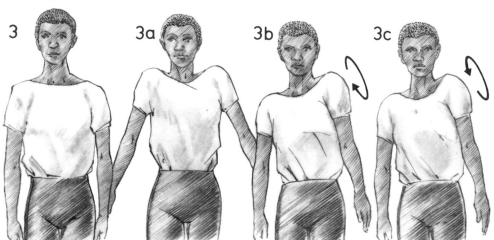

4 Arms and shoulders

Stand as for exercise 1. Raise your arms to the sides at shoulder level, bending your elbows and touching your shoulders with your hands (**a**). Keeping your elbows bent, pull your left arm up (**b**). Lower it and repeat with your right arm (**c**).

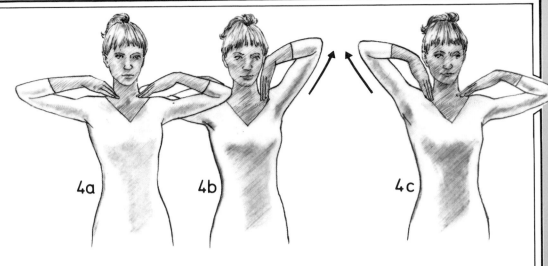

4a   4b   4c

5 Legs and abdomen

Lie flat on your back. Stretch your legs out hard for a few seconds, pointing your toes (**a**), then let them go limp. Bend your left foot at the ankle as if you were trying to bring your toes toward your shin (**b**). Keeping your foot in this position and your leg straight, lift your leg about 15cm off the ground (**c**). Hold this position for a few seconds, then lower your leg and relax it. Repeat with the other leg. Only your legs should be tensed during this exercise: keep the rest of your body as relaxed as possible.

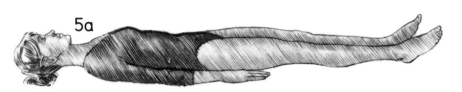

5a

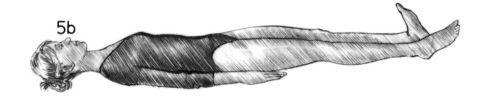

5b

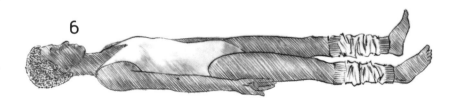

5c

6 Total relaxation

Lie flat on your back, feet slightly apart, arms slightly away from your body, palms upwards. Cover yourself with a blanket if you feel at all cold. Close your eyes. Breathe deeply and evenly, without making any effort to expand and contract your chest. Think of something pleasant and undemanding – a flower, a colour, a piece of music. Remain in this position for about 10 minutes, then open your eyes, roll onto your side, and get up slowly and gradually.

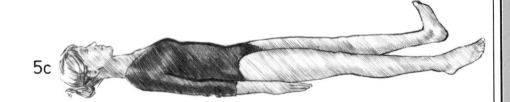

6

©DIAGRAM

Sleep

Sleep is vital for your body and mind to remain in good health, although an occasional sleepless night will not do you very much harm. We all need sleep to keep us alive, just as we need food and water. If we have more than one or two sleepless nights in a row, it affects how we look and feel. Eyes, hair, and skin look dull and lifeless, muscles become tense, and we lack concentration and coordination. Severe sleep deprivation can lead to major personality changes and disorders.

What happens when you sleep?

You spend about three-quarters of the time you are asleep in a deep sleep called orthodox sleep. This is when your body is at its most relaxed. Your heartbeat slows, your blood pressure is lowered, and your damaged body tissues are being replaced.

The other quarter of your sleeping time is spent in paradoxical (REM) sleep. This is when you dream. Although your eyes are closed, there is rapid eye movement (REM) behind the lids. Your heartbeat and breathing become irregular, and your brain is as active as it is when you are awake. Periods of paradoxical sleep alternate with periods of orthodox sleep, and both are essential for your health. Everybody dreams (even those of us who are unaware of dreaming): people who are deprived of paradoxical (REM) sleep can easily become emotionally disturbed.

How much sleep do you need?

People vary in the amount of sleep they need. On average, an adult needs about seven hours sleep in a 24 hour period, but some people will feel refreshed after only 2–3 hours sleep, while others will need 9–10 hours. As you get older, you usually need less sleep than when you were younger. You are also more likely to sleep for several short periods, rather than taking one long rest.

Do you sleep well?

Many people wake up in the morning feeling unrefreshed and as if they have hardly slept at all. In fact they have probably had more sleep than they think – research has shown that most insomniacs are getting only 40 minutes less sleep than "normal" sleepers. If you have problems getting to sleep, staying asleep, or getting enough sleep, take a look at the amount of stress in your life. Reducing your stress level will help you to sleep better. But as sleeping badly can make you stressed, you also need to tackle your sleep problem at the same time.

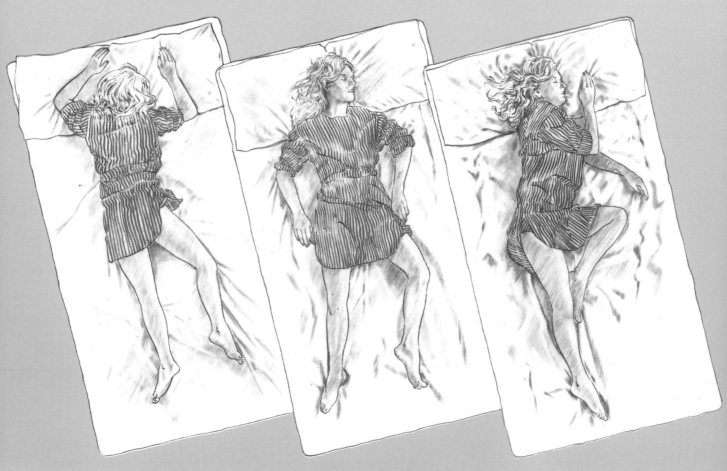

HELPING YOURSELF SLEEP

Make sure that your bed is comfortable and provides firm but even support for your body.

Make sure that your bedroom is comfortable – neither too hot nor too cold, well ventilated, and so on.

Most people sleep better in the dark: if your curtains let in too much light, try wearing a sleep mask.

Noise may keep you awake: consider secondary glazing for your windows or try wearing earplugs. Remember that ticking clocks and other household noises can be as disturbing as road, rail, and airport noises.

As far as possible, match your sleep periods to your natural body rhythms. If you are a night person, you will have problems if you try to force yourself to go to bed early and to get up early. If you are a morning person, you will probably wake up early even when you go to bed late.

Because your body works on a 24 hour cycle, you will probably find it easier to get to sleep if you establish a regular routine, i.e. going to bed and getting up at roughly the same time each day.

Start winding down about an hour before you go to bed. Avoid strenuous exercise or drinking stimulants, as these will make you feel wide awake. Similarly, don't become involved in intellectually stimulating tasks just before you go to bed.

If you cannot sleep, don't lie in bed worrying about it. Make yourself a warm drink, read a book, or listen to the radio instead. Accept the fact that you are awake and you will probably fall asleep!

Think carefully before taking sleeping pills. Used for a short, limited period they can have their place in helping you over a difficult time, but in the long term they will do nothing to solve the problem of why you are not sleeping well. Sleeping pills also suppress REM sleep, and so can leave you feeling tired and washed out in the morning, instead of feeling refreshed.

Sleeping positions
During sleep we move our bodies into a variety of different positions. In general, the more we spread our limbs, the more relaxed we feel. Fetal or semi-fetal positions often suggest tension or insecurity.

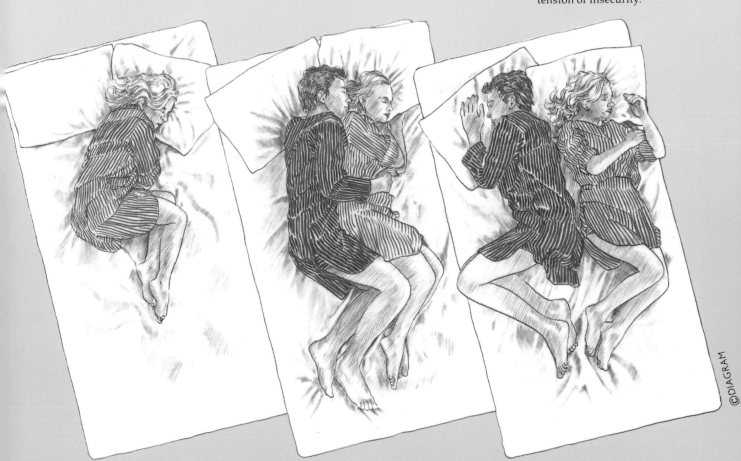

©DIAGRAM

37

Massage

Massage is a very effective way to reduce stress and tension. It stretches and relaxes the fibres of the muscles, making them more supple and increasing the blood flow to the area. This improved blood flow helps to remove the waste products and impurities that collect in stiff muscles. And because it leaves you feeling physically relaxed, a good massage will leave you feeling mentally relaxed as well.

You have several choices when it comes to massage. You can go to a professional masseuse for treatment, ask a friend to massage you (and then massage him or her in exchange), or even massage yourself. And you can choose from several different types of massage – reflexology, for example, in which only the feet are massaged, or shiatsu, a Japanese form of massage performed almost entirely with the pad of the thumb. The most usual type of massage for relaxation is described here. It is based on Swedish massage, and uses a wide variety of strokes with different parts of the hands and with different amounts of pressure.

MASSAGE STROKES

If you have a professional massage, you will find that the masseuse uses a number of different manipulative techniques, called strokes. The basic stroke is a stroking movement, with the hands gliding over your skin. The masseuse will fit her hands to the contours of your muscles and then move them over your skin with differing amounts of pressure, depending on how tense you are.

1 Stroking movements
2 Kneading movements
3 Friction
4 Percussion movements

Kneading movements, in which the muscles are gently lifted, wrung, and squeezed, are used to stimulate the blood supply. Friction – massaging in small circles using the pads of the fingers, the thumb, or the heel of the hand – is used where work is needed on "knots" in the deep tissues. Percussion movements (including hacking, tapping, slapping, and pinching) are used to stimulate, rather than relax, the system.

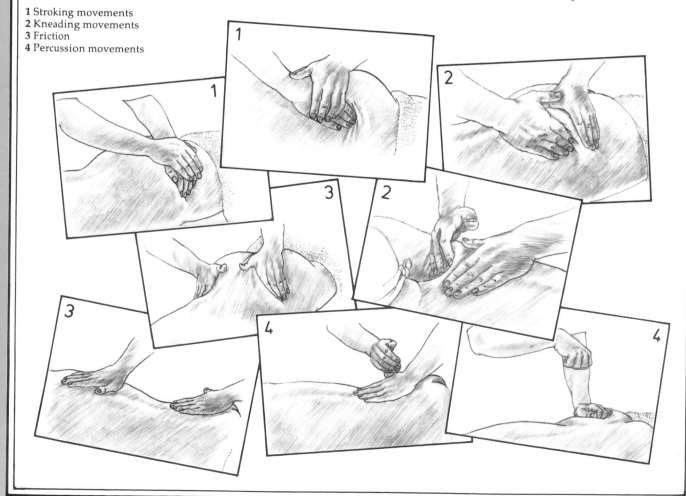

HOME MASSAGE

You need very little equipment for a home massage. If you have a large, sturdy table, cover it with towels or a blanket, and use it as a massage table. If not, spread out your towels or blanket on the floor. Don't use a bed for massage: however hard the bed, it will still be too soft for the massage to be effective.

Make sure that the room is warm and that the lighting is soft. Try to avoid being disturbed, and switch off the telephone. If you are giving the massage, make sure that your nails are short and that your hands are warm. You will need some oil to use as a lubricant to avoid friction. Special perfumed massage oils are available, but a bland vegetable cooking oil will be just as effective. Never pour the oil directly onto the skin of the person you are massaging. Warm it first by pouring it into your hand and rubbing it between your palms. The person who is being massaged should preferably be naked. Use a towel or blanket to cover the parts of the body that are not being worked on to prevent them getting cold.

Massage should always be done gently. Use even pressure and take care when you are working on the less protected parts of the body, such as the abdomen and the kidney area. Once you have started a massage, try to keep at least one hand in contact with the person being massaged until you have finished. And use your own body carefully when you are giving a massage: make sure that you do not strain your back.

Full body massage
This is a simple programme of massage for the whole body, using the basic stroking movement.
1 With your hands parallel to each other, stroke down the front of the body and up the sides.

2 Place your hands parallel to each other on either side of the spine. Stroke downward to the buttocks and then upward round the sides of the body.

3 Starting at the shoulder, stroke down the front of the arm, then up the back of it.

4 Starting at the thigh, stroke down the front of the leg, then up the back of it.

5 Place the palms of the hands over the eyes, covering the face. Stroke outward with both hands at the same time.

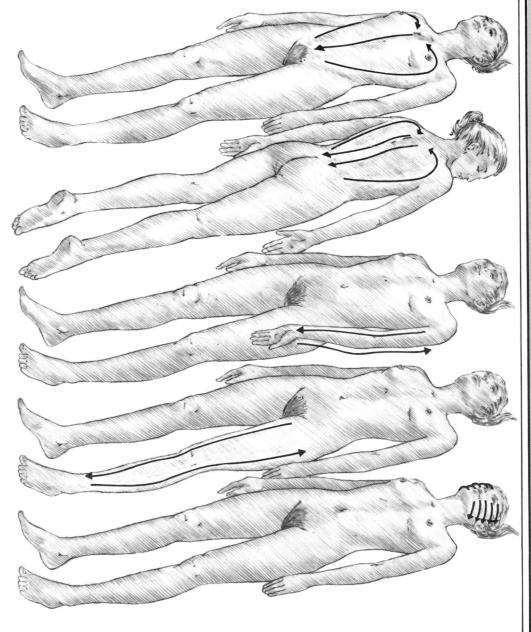

©DIAGRAM

39

Exercise

Our bodies are designed for exercise. Without exercise our muscles gradually weaken, our joints stiffen, and our hearts and lungs function less efficiently. Unfit people tend to tire easily and to lack energy and enthusiasm for life. An unfit woman can only make use of about 30% of her body's total energy capacity: it is not surprising that an average day's routine leaves her feeling exhausted, with nothing left to spare. A fit woman, on the other hand, only needs part of her energy to get through an average day: she has about 30% of her total energy capacity left with which to enjoy herself.

If you deny yourself exercise, you are denying yourself the chance to get the most out of life. Exercise will make you stronger and more supple, improve your posture and your circulation, burn up the excess fats in your system, improve your digestion, increase the capacity of your lungs, and make your heart stronger. You will sleep better, and feel more relaxed and less stressed. Best of all, you will look better – exercise is one of the best and simplest beauty routines you can adopt.

CHOOSING YOUR FORM OF EXERCISE

On the following pages we describe some of the many forms of exercise that are available today. How should you choose between them?

First of all, remember that exercise should be a pleasure, not a punishment. Choose a form of exercise that you enjoy, or you will soon be finding an excuse to give it up!

Secondly, think about your personal needs and your lifestyle. Is there a particular part of your body you want to improve? What facilities for sports are there near you? How much time each week can you spend exercising? Would you prefer to exercise on your own or to work in a group?

Thirdly, think about your body type. Research has shown that certain body types are more suited to some sports and forms of exercise than to others. This information is summarised in table **A**. Finally, remember that for total fitness your personal exercise plan should include three basic essentials: strength exercises, suppleness exercises, and stamina exercises. Strength exercises give shape to your body muscles, and prepare your body to cope with any situations that need extra effort; suppleness exercises keep your body flexible, loosen stiff joints, and help you move gracefully; stamina exercises improve the performance of your heart and lungs. Use the summary in table **B** to help you choose complementary exercises that will give you the best all-round results.

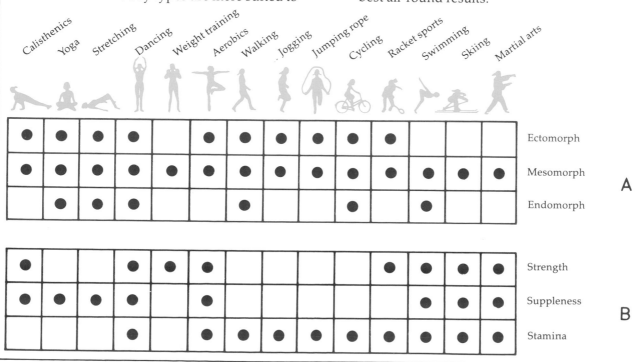

Table A

	Calisthenics	Yoga	Stretching	Dancing	Weight training	Aerobics	Walking	Jogging	Jumping rope	Cycling	Racket sports	Swimming	Skiing	Martial arts
Ectomorph	●	●	●	●		●	●	●	●	●	●			
Mesomorph	●	●	●	●	●	●	●	●	●	●	●	●	●	●
Endomorph		●	●	●		●				●		●		

Table B

	Calisthenics	Yoga	Stretching	Dancing	Weight training	Aerobics	Walking	Jogging	Jumping rope	Cycling	Racket sports	Swimming	Skiing	Martial arts
Strength	●			●	●	●					●	●	●	●
Suppleness	●	●	●	●		●						●	●	●
Stamina				●		●	●	●	●	●	●	●	●	●

EXERCISING SAFELY

When you first start exercising, start gently and build up your level of fitness gradually. If you are very unfit, begin by increasing the amount of activity in your daily life – walk instead of taking the car, use the stairs instead of the lift, and so on. As you become fitter, you can start on your chosen exercise plan, taking it slowly at first, and progressing more vigorously as your strength, suppleness, and stamina increase. Trying to do too much too soon will simply leave you exhausted, aching, and discouraged, and at risk from strains, sprains, and other more serious muscle damage. Never try to push yourself beyond your limits, or to force your body into painful positions. Whatever form of exercise you choose, always begin each session by warming up and end it by cooling down, or you will be inviting muscle strains and soreness. A selection of warm-up exercises are given on pp. 42–43.

While you exercise, watch out for warning signs that something may be wrong. Stop exercising at once if you experience any of the symptoms in the table below, and consult your doctor if they are severe or persistent.

A simple pulse test will show you if you are exercising safely. Add a handicap figure of 40 to your age, and take this number from 200. This is your maximum safe pulse rate. As soon as you begin to feel tired and breathless, take your pulse. If your pulse rate is above your maximum safety figure, stop exercising, and rest. As you get fitter, reduce your handicap figure by units of 10 until you have removed it altogether. If you are over 45, reduce your handicap by units of 5 to a minimum of 20.

Warning signs
- Dizziness, light-headedness, confusion, or fainting
- Irregular pulse, palpitations, unusual pressure or pain in the chest, arm, or throat
- Cold sweats
- Extreme breathlessness
- Cramp or stitch
- Nausea or vomiting
- Joint or muscle pain
- Any other abnormal body response

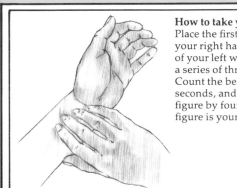

How to take your pulse
Place the first three fingers of your right hand on the inside of your left wrist. You will feel a series of throbs or beats. Count the beats for 15 seconds, and multiply this figure by four. This final figure is your pulse rate.

HOW MUCH EXERCISE

Research shows that fairly short exercise sessions every day or every other day are more beneficial than a long session once a week. Start by exercising for 5–10 minutes three times a week, and gradually build up the number and length of your exercise sessions. For total fitness you should aim for three 20–30 minute sessions of stamina exercises each week, plus one or two sessions of strength and suppleness exercises.

WHEN TO EXERCISE

You can exercise at any time of day that suits your personal routine and your body rhythm, as long as you are not exercising on a full stomach (leave at least an hour between a meal and an exercise session). Morning exercise can be an excellent way to wake up, and it has the advantage of leaving the rest of the day free. You will need to warm up your muscles carefully if you plan to exercise as soon as you have got out of bed. Exercising before lunch can be a useful break during the middle of the day, and can help to prevent afternoon tiredness and boredom. Evening exercise will help you to relax and get rid of the day's tensions. Allow yourself plenty of time between your exercise session and going to bed, or your body will be too stimulated for you to fall asleep easily.

WHAT TO WEAR

You can wear whatever you like to exercise in, as long as you feel comfortable and can move easily and freely. Choose either loose, non-restrictive clothing, such as a track suit, or clothes that will stretch with you, such as a leotard. If you feel conspicuous in a leotard because you are out of shape, try wearing a cheerful baggy T-shirt over a pair of tights. Cotton clothes will "breathe" as you sweat; you may find them more comfortable than synthetics which may make you feel sticky. Remember that you will need a sweater or jacket and perhaps a pair of leg-warmers to keep you warm when you finish your exercise session. A towelling sweatband will help to keep your hair out of your face. Most indoor exercises can be performed in bare feet or in flat, soft, non-slip shoes. Outdoor exercise and most sports need special shoes – you will damage your feet and legs if you start running in the wrong shoes, for example. Information about any special clothing or footwear needed for a particular form of exercise are included in the descriptions on the following pages.

Warming up

Warm-up exercises are gentle exercises that loosen your muscles, raise your body temperature, increase your heart and breathing rate, and generally prepare your body for more intensive forms of exercise. If you start exercising without warming up you run the risk of pulling a muscle or of more serious injury. A 5 or 10 minute warm-up session can save you days or even weeks of pain.

Cooling down is as important as warming up. When you suddenly stop exercising without cooling down, your circulation slows down too quickly to allow your body to deal with the waste products that your muscles have been producing while you were exercising. A 5 or 10 minute cooling down session will keep your blood circulating fast enough to get rid of nearly all of the waste products, and will also let your body temperature and heart and breathing rates reduce gradually.

The exercises on these pages can be used for both warming up and cooling down. However, when you are cooling down you may wish to replace running on the spot by 1–2 minutes of walking around breathing deeply.

1 Neck circles
Stand upright with your feet shoulder width apart and your hands hanging loosely by your sides. Drop your chin onto your chest (**a**), then roll your head round to the left (**b**), round to the back (**c**), round to the right (**d**), and then round to your chest again in a complete circle. Then reverse direction circling to the right. Repeat three times in each direction.

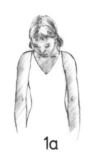
1a

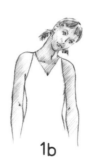
1b

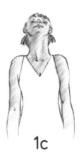
1c

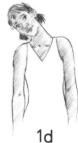
1d

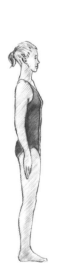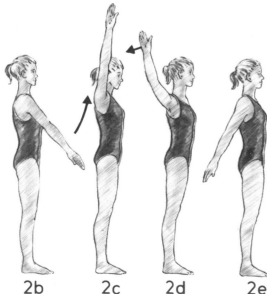
2a 2b 2c 2d 2e

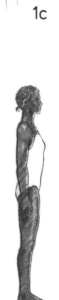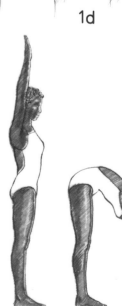
3a b 3c

2 Arm circling
Stand upright with your feet shoulder width apart (**a**). Swing both arms forward (**b**) and upward (**c**), then take them backward (**d**) and down (**e**), making large circles. Then reverse the action, circling the arms in the opposite direction. Repeat up to 20 times each way.

3 Touching toes
Stand upright with your feet together (**a**). Stretch your arms above your head (**b**), then bend down as far as possible, reaching down to touch the ground in front of your toes (**c**). Bob gently, then straighten up into the starting position. Repeat up to 10 times.

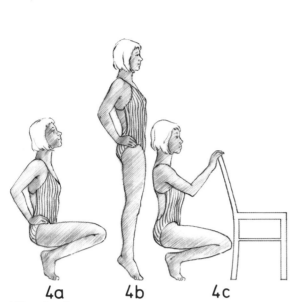

4a **4b** **4c**

5a **5b** **5c**

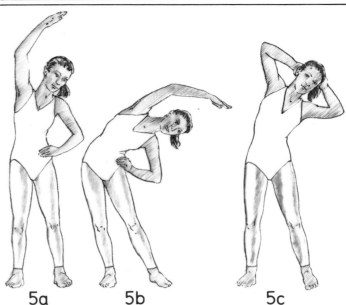

4 Knee bends
Stand upright with your feet together, toes turned out, and hands on hips. Sink down into a squat, keeping your back straight (**a**). Straighten your legs and rise up onto your toes (**b**). Repeat five times.
When you first try this exercise you may find it helpful to rest your hands on the back of a chair to help you keep your balance (**c**). If possible you should keep your feet flat on the floor when you squat, but you may find it easier if you rise up on your toes.

5 Body bends
Stand upright with your feet shoulder width apart. Place your left hand on your hip, and curve your right hand above your head (**a**). Bend slowly to your left side as far as you can (**b**), then bob gently. Change arms and repeat to the other side. Repeat up to five times on each side. This exercise can also be performed with both hands clasped behind your head (**c**).

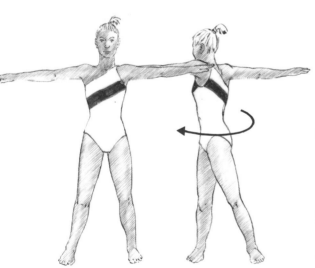

6a **6b**

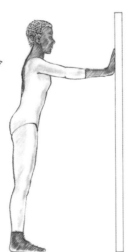

7a **7b**

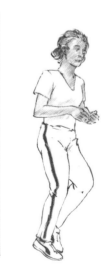

8

6 Body twists
Stand upright with your feet shoulder width apart. Stretch your arms out to the side, palms down (**a**). Twist your body to the right as far as possible (**b**), then to the left. Repeat five times to each side.

7 Calf stretches
Stand about .91m from a wall, with your feet together and your hands resting flat on the wall (**a**). Lean forward, bending your arms and keeping your heels on the floor (**b**). (If you cannot feel a slight stretch in your calf muscles, you need to stand farther away from the wall.)

Hold this position for about 15 seconds, and then use your arms to push yourself upright. Repeat five times.

8 Running on the spot
Run gently on the spot for about 1 minute, raising your feet at least 10cm from the floor and landing on the balls of your feet.

Calisthenics

Calisthenics are exercises that involve rhythmic, repetitive movements. They will help you strengthen your muscles (and so improve the shape of your body) and make you more supple. They are not stamina exercises, and so to be fully fit you must supplement them with some form of exercise that strengthens your heart and lungs. Like any other form of exercise, calisthenics have both advantages and drawbacks: these are summarised in the table right.

HOW TO EXERCISE

Calisthenic exercises must be performed rhythmically, and you will probably find it easier and more enjoyable to do them to music. For maximum benefit, each exercise needs to be repeated 30 times without a break. Start with five repetitions of each exercise, and gradually build up to the full 30. Pause between exercises, but try not to stop and rest. Instead, walk on the spot or around the room for about a minute. This will help to keep up your metabolic rate and make the exercises more effective. Once you can perform the full number of repetitions easily, increase the speed with which you do them. Most of the warm-up exercises shown on pp. 42–43 can be used as part of your calisthenics session. Once you have warmed up, perform them again more vigorously, building up to 30 repetitions of each. Combined with the exercises shown here they will form a full calisthenics session. Remember to cool down when you have finished exercising.

Advantages
- Easy to learn
- Need no special equipment
- Need very little space
- Suitable indoors or outdoors
- Can be used to exercise all major muscles
- Can be performed alone or in a group
- Improve strength and suppleness

Disadvantages
- Must be supplemented by stamina exercises
- Number of repetitions required can lead to boredom

EXERCISE PROGRAMMES

Instead of planning your own calisthenics session, you may prefer to follow a formal exercise programme. These programmes are carefully planned to include exercises for all parts of your body. They remove any guesswork from becoming progressively fitter – you begin at the most basic level of the programme, and gradually progress to more demanding levels at set intervals. Following a programme means that you are less likely to overextend yourself in an initial burst of enthusiasm, and many people enjoy the challenge of reaching a set target. The Royal Canadian Air Force 5BX and XBX programmes are probably the best known, but several others are commercially available, and the United States and many other national governments publish their own programmes. Check carefully before you choose a programme. Some include full details of warming up, cooling down, and supplementary stamina exercises, while others concentrate exclusively on the details of the calisthenics session.

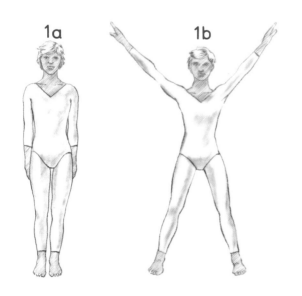

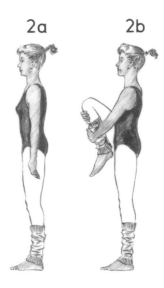

1 Jumping jacks
Stand upright, feet together, and hands by your sides (**a**). Jump up and land with your feet apart, swinging your arms out to the side and up so that your body forms an X (**b**). Jump back into the starting position and repeat.

2 Knee pulls
Stand upright with your feet together and your arms by your sides (**a**). Raise your right knee as high as you can. Grasp your right knee with both hands and pull it toward your chest (**b**). Keep your head up and your back straight. Lower your right leg and repeat with your left leg.

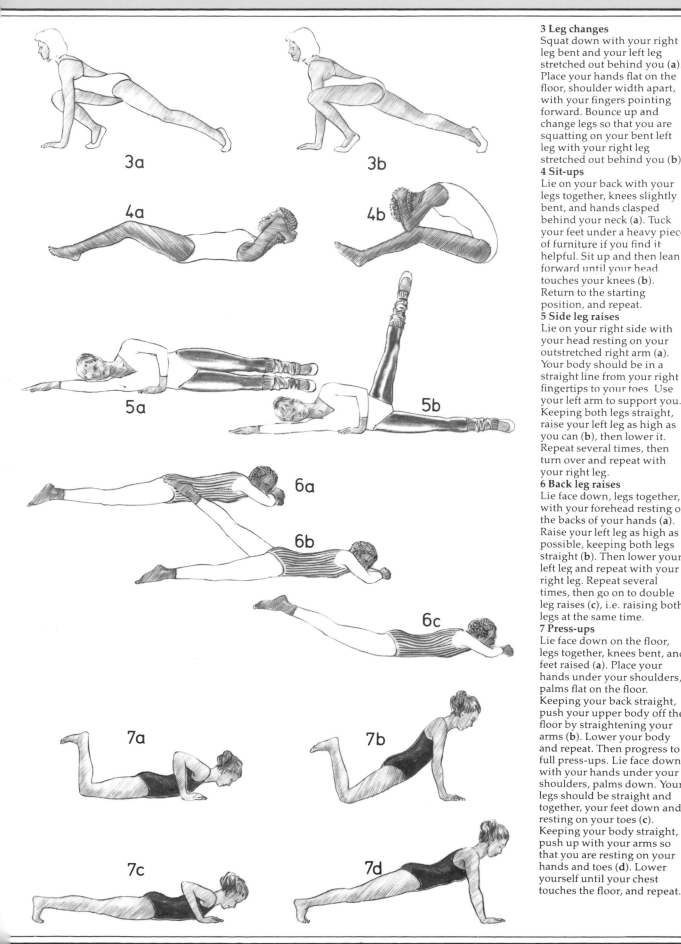

3 Leg changes
Squat down with your right leg bent and your left leg stretched out behind you (**a**). Place your hands flat on the floor, shoulder width apart, with your fingers pointing forward. Bounce up and change legs so that you are squatting on your bent left leg with your right leg stretched out behind you (**b**).

4 Sit-ups
Lie on your back with your legs together, knees slightly bent, and hands clasped behind your neck (**a**). Tuck your feet under a heavy piece of furniture if you find it helpful. Sit up and then lean forward until your head touches your knees (**b**). Return to the starting position, and repeat.

5 Side leg raises
Lie on your right side with your head resting on your outstretched right arm (**a**). Your body should be in a straight line from your right fingertips to your toes. Use your left arm to support you. Keeping both legs straight, raise your left leg as high as you can (**b**), then lower it. Repeat several times, then turn over and repeat with your right leg.

6 Back leg raises
Lie face down, legs together, with your forehead resting on the backs of your hands (**a**). Raise your left leg as high as possible, keeping both legs straight (**b**). Then lower your left leg and repeat with your right leg. Repeat several times, then go on to double leg raises (**c**), i.e. raising both legs at the same time.

7 Press-ups
Lie face down on the floor, legs together, knees bent, and feet raised (**a**). Place your hands under your shoulders, palms flat on the floor. Keeping your back straight, push your upper body off the floor by straightening your arms (**b**). Lower your body and repeat. Then progress to full press-ups. Lie face down with your hands under your shoulders, palms down. Your legs should be straight and together, your feet down and resting on your toes (**c**). Keeping your body straight, push up with your arms so that you are resting on your hands and toes (**d**). Lower yourself until your chest touches the floor, and repeat.

Yoga

Yoga is an ancient Indian philosophy that exists in many different forms. The form that is most popular in the Western world and which is the most useful as a form of exercise is Hatha (physical) yoga. Hatha yoga combines a variety of postures or poses called ansanas with breathing exercises to have an effect on all parts of the body. The ansanas are unequaled in improving suppleness, and because yoga places a great deal of emphasis on the strength and flexibility of the spine, they will also help you to improve your posture. The breathing exercises are designed to increase the amount of oxygen in your body. The combination of ansanas and breathing exercises can counteract stress, reduce tension, and promote a general feeling of well-being.

The ansanas shown on these pages can all be learned easily and practiced at home without supervision. If you decide you would like to make yoga a regular part of your exercise programme, you will probably find it worthwhile to go to a class. A properly qualified teacher will be able to show you exactly how each ansana should be performed, as well as teaching you the specialised yoga breathing exercises. A class will also be useful if you are interested in learning more about the philosophy of yoga and yoga meditation.

HOW TO EXERCISE

You can practice yoga in any quiet, well-ventilated area that has enough floor space to allow you to stretch comfortably in all directions. Move slowly and rhythmically into each pose, and then hold your position, remaining absolutely motionless. At first you should try to hold each pose for about 10 seconds. As you become more proficient, gradually increase the time to 15–20 seconds. Your breathing should be steady and rhythmic throughout each ansana. Relax completely between poses for 10–15 seconds.

You will almost certainly find some ansanas easier than others, depending on your individual build and flexibility. Never force your body into any of the poses that you find difficult: go just as far as you can, and stop as soon as you feel any strain. Your suppleness will improve with regular practice, and you will soon be able to go on to the next stage.

1 Tadasana (basic standing pose)
Stand with your feet together, your weight evenly on heels and toes. Keep your head up, chin tucked in, spine stretched, and knees pulled up. Your buttock and stomach muscles should be tightened. Your shoulders, arms, and hands should be relaxed and loose.

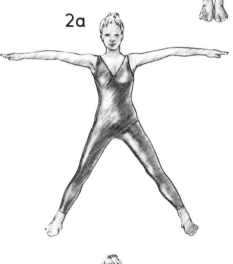

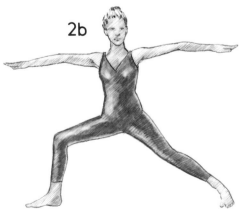

2 Virabhadrasana (warrior pose)
Stand in the basic standing pose. Jump so that your feet are about 1.2m apart, with your arms stretched out at shoulder level, palms down (**a**). Turn your right foot out so that it is at right angles to your left foot. Bend your right leg, aiming to have your thigh and lower leg at right angles to each other, with your knee directly over your ankle (**b**). Hold this position. Return slowly to the standing position and repeat to the other side.

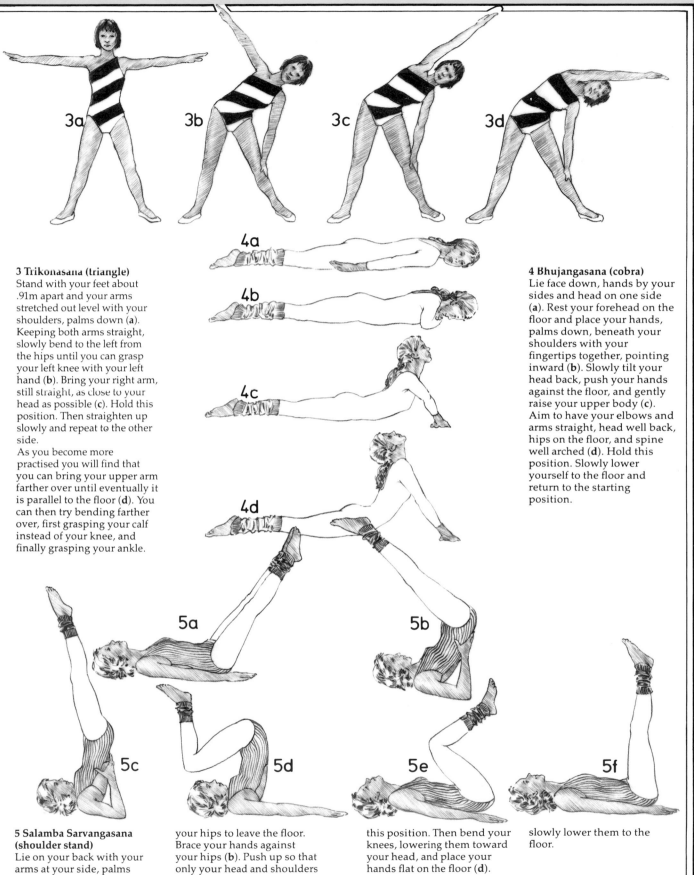

3 Trikonasana (triangle)

Stand with your feet about .91m apart and your arms stretched out level with your shoulders, palms down (**a**). Keeping both arms straight, slowly bend to the left from the hips until you can grasp your left knee with your left hand (**b**). Bring your right arm, still straight, as close to your head as possible (**c**). Hold this position. Then straighten up slowly and repeat to the other side.

As you become more practised you will find that you can bring your upper arm farther over until eventually it is parallel to the floor (**d**). You can then try bending farther over, first grasping your calf instead of your knee, and finally grasping your ankle.

4 Bhujangasana (cobra)

Lie face down, hands by your sides and head on one side (**a**). Rest your forehead on the floor and place your hands, palms down, beneath your shoulders with your fingertips together, pointing inward (**b**). Slowly tilt your head back, push your hands against the floor, and gently raise your upper body (**c**). Aim to have your elbows and arms straight, head well back, hips on the floor, and spine well arched (**d**). Hold this position. Slowly lower yourself to the floor and return to the starting position.

5 Salamba Sarvangasana (shoulder stand)

Lie on your back with your arms at your side, palms down. Keeping your legs together, slowly raise your legs (**a**), swinging them up with enough momentum for your hips to leave the floor. Brace your hands against your hips (**b**). Push up so that only your head and shoulders are on the floor and your back is supported on your hands (**c**). Your chin should be tucked into your chest. Hold this position. Then bend your knees, lowering them toward your head, and place your hands flat on the floor (**d**). Roll forward, keeping your knees bent until your hips touch the floor (**e**). Then straighten your legs (**f**) and slowly lower them to the floor.

Stretching

Stretching is a very natural form of exercise. We instinctively stretch when we wake up and get out of bed in the morning, and feel more awake and able to move more easily as a result. Unless joints and muscles are stretched regularly, their tissues soon lose their elasticity and become stiff – and stiff joints and muscles can soon become sore joints and muscles. Stretching exercises help to loosen joints and muscles, reduce tension, and relieve aches and pains. Practised regularly, they will make you more supple, especially if your favourite sport or form of exercise is one that has a tightening effect on your muscles.

HOW TO EXERCISE

Move gently into position until you feel an easy stretch in your muscles. Hold this position for 20–30 seconds. Then stretch a little farther, so that you feel a greater pull in your muscles, and hold this position for another 30 seconds. Never stretch so far that the stretch causes pain – you will then be straining your muscles instead of stretching. Always hold the stretch without moving: never bounce. Breathe normally and rhythmically as you exercise. If the stretch involves bending forward, breathe out as you bend, breathe normally while you hold the stretch, and breathe in as you straighten up.

1 This stretch will help your waist, hips, stomach, and back.
Lie flat on your back and extend your arms over your head, palms up. Stretch your right arm and right leg while keeping the whole of your left side relaxed. Hold the stretch. Then relax and repeat with your left arm and leg.

2 This stretch is good for your back and shoulders.
Lie on your back with your knees bent, feet apart and flat on the floor, hands by your sides, palms down (**a**). Push down on your hands and feet and gradually lift your back off the floor until your body is resting on your head, shoulders, arms, hands, and feet (**b**). Hold the stretch.

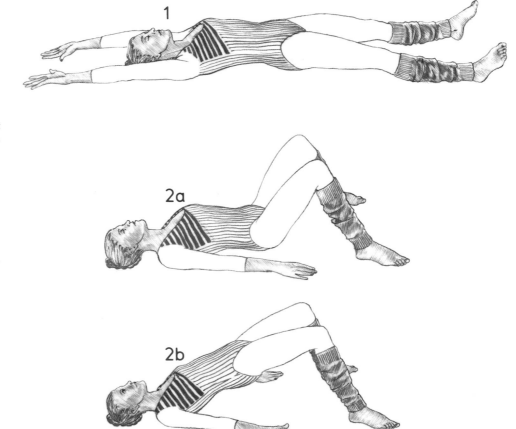

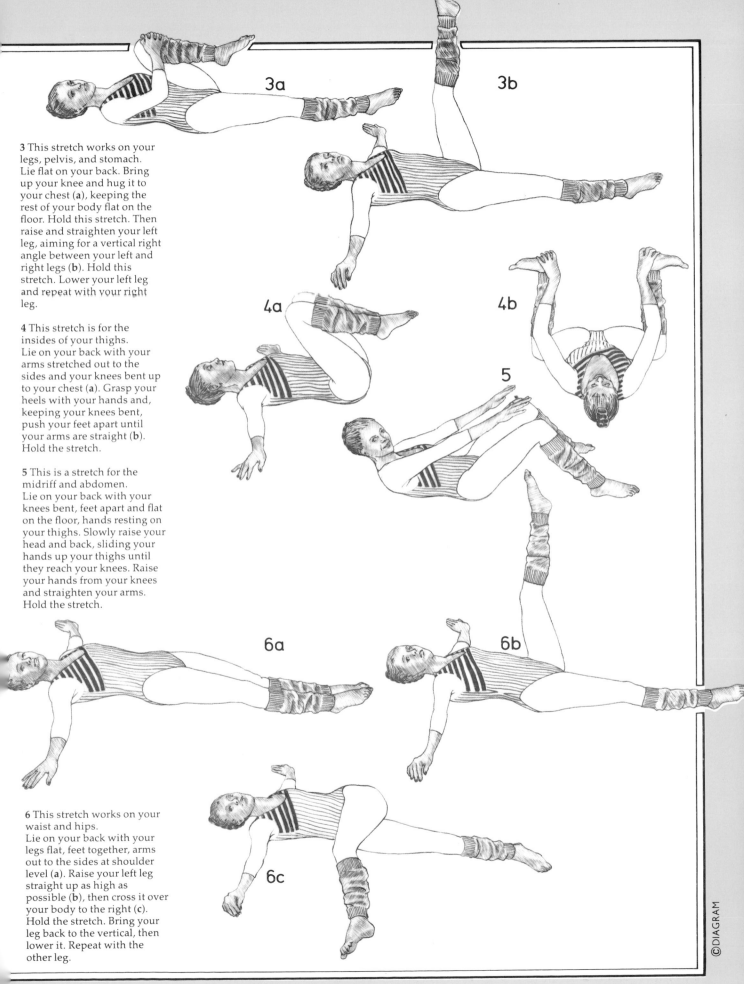

3 This stretch works on your legs, pelvis, and stomach. Lie flat on your back. Bring up your knee and hug it to your chest (**a**), keeping the rest of your body flat on the floor. Hold this stretch. Then raise and straighten your left leg, aiming for a vertical right angle between your left and right legs (**b**). Hold this stretch. Lower your left leg and repeat with your right leg.

4 This stretch is for the insides of your thighs. Lie on your back with your arms stretched out to the sides and your knees bent up to your chest (**a**). Grasp your heels with your hands and, keeping your knees bent, push your feet apart until your arms are straight (**b**). Hold the stretch.

5 This is a stretch for the midriff and abdomen. Lie on your back with your knees bent, feet apart and flat on the floor, hands resting on your thighs. Slowly raise your head and back, sliding your hands up your thighs until they reach your knees. Raise your hands from your knees and straighten your arms. Hold the stretch.

6 This stretch works on your waist and hips. Lie on your back with your legs flat, feet together, arms out to the sides at shoulder level (**a**). Raise your left leg straight up as high as possible (**b**), then cross it over your body to the right (**c**). Hold the stretch. Bring your leg back to the vertical, then lower it. Repeat with the other leg.

©DIAGRAM

Dance

Ballet, tap, jazz, modern, disco, folk, country, square, Latin-American – there's a type of dancing to suit all tastes. There are also exercise programmes, such as Dancercise and Jazzercise, which are based on dance movements. All of them are excellent all-round forms of exercise, as they help to develop strength, suppleness, and stamina. Consider your taste in music when you are deciding which type of dance to take up. For example, if you enjoy rock music and dislike folk music, you will probably prefer jazz dancing or disco to any of the many types of country or folk dancing. You will also need to think about your life style and the way in which you like to exercise. Disco, Latin-American, folk, country, and square dancing can all form part of your social life: you can enjoy an evening at a dance with your friends and get all the benefits of exercising at the same time. Ballet, jazz, tap, and modern dance will

probably involve you in regular classes, but once you have learned the basic skills you can practise them at home on your own. You can disco dance alone or in company, but you will obviously need a partner for Latin-American, and probably a group of eight people for most types of country and folk dancing. If you are interested in a type of dance that you have not tried before, ask your local dance centre, school, or society if you can join in a beginner's class for a week or two so that you can see if it's the right one for you.

Whichever form of dance you choose, you will find that practising the ballet-based exercises shown here will help you improve your dancing. They are also a useful supplement to social dancing or to dancing that needs a group of people as they can be practised at home on your own. To do them you will need something to hold on to – a rail or the back of a chair at roughly waist height.

1 Waist stretch
Stand holding the rail with one hand (**a**), heels together, toes turned out, free arm curved above your head. Bend backward (**b**), keeping your free arm extended. Pull over toward the rail (**c**), then pull your body forward and down toward the floor,

keeping your stomach well in. Bend forward from your hips (**d**), letting your free hand brush the floor, and keeping your knees tight, back straight, and stomach in. Raise your upper body from the hips until it is at right angles to your legs (**e**), keeping your free arm

extended. Then return to the starting position. Repeat up to 10 times, then turn around and repeat up to 10 times on the other side.

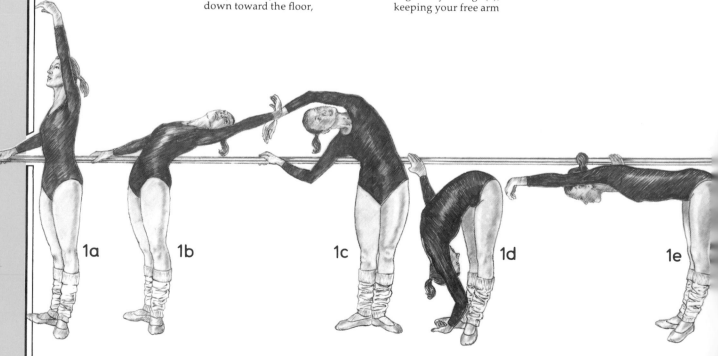

1a 1b 1c 1d 1e

WHAT TO WEAR

What you wear depends on the type of dance you choose. For ballet, jazz, and modern dance you will need a leotard and tights. Jazz and modern dancers often dance in bare feet, but for ballet you will need proper ballet shoes, with or without blocks depending on your level of skill. For most other forms of dance you can wear whatever you feel comfortable in, but – apart from Latin-American and disco – you may well need special shoes. Tap dancers usually wear medium-heeled strap shoes with metal taps fixed to the soles. Shoes for country and folk dancing vary, depending on the type of dancing involved and its country of origin. Take a pair of sneakers or other soft shoes along to your first folk or country class in case your everyday shoes are not suitable, and ask other members of the class for advice on the best type of shoe to buy if you decide to take it up on a regular basis.

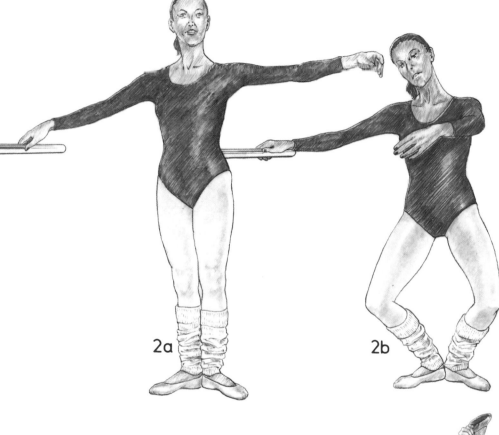

2 Demi plié
Stand holding the rail with one hand (**a**). Your heels should be together and your toes turned out. Keep your back straight, stomach in, and legs and knees pulled up. Extend your free arm out to the side, keeping it slightly bent at the elbow. Now bend at the knees, letting your knees push out over your feet (**b**). Keep your back straight, head up, and feet flat on the floor. As you bend, bring your free arm round in front of you. Return to the starting position and repeat up to 10 times.
When you are comfortable with the demi plié, go on to the grand plié. Begin as for a demi plié, but bend your knees farther so that you are in a deep squat with your knees turned out over your feet and your heels off the ground. Return to the starting position and repeat up to 10 times.

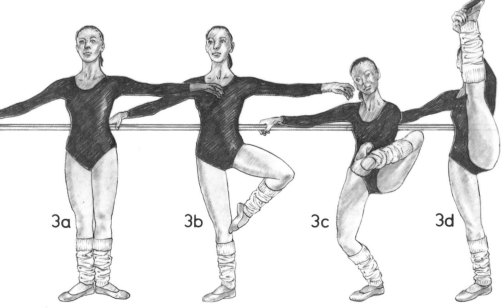

3 Leg stretch
Stand holding the rail with one hand (**a**), heels together, toes turned out, and free arm extended at shoulder level. Bring the foot farthest from the rail up to knee height (**b**), turning your bent knee out and pointing your toe. Bend your supporting leg and take hold of your raised foot near the heel (**c**). Straighten both legs (**d**). Keep both legs straight as you return to the starting position. Repeat up to five times, then turn around and repeat up to five times with the other leg.

Weight training

Don't confuse weight training with weight lifting! If you follow a weight training programme you will not be straining to lift heavy weights but carrying out a series of repeated, rhythmic exercises with light weights of 2–6lb. Weight training works on the principle of passive resistance – the more resistance your muscles have to work against, the stronger they become. Weights provide the increased resistance necessary to develop strong muscles. In fact, weight training is one of the fastest and best ways to improve your muscle strength and your figure. You can use it to tone up specific sets of muscles or to reshape parts of your body which you would like to change. Weight training will not give you enormous "body-builder's" muscles: it is physically impossible for women to develop muscles of such size. Remember that although working with weights is unequaled as a strength exercise, it will do nothing for your suppleness or stamina, so you will need to supplement it with other types of exercise for all-round fitness.

EQUIPMENT
When you first try weight training, improvise the weights from objects that you have around the house. Use cans of food or bags of sugar for hand-held weights, and a broom handle or length of wood as a barbell substitute. If you decide to follow a complete weight training programme, you will need a pair of dumbells, a barbell, and a pair of strap-on ankle weights. A dumbell is a short bar with a weight fixed at each end: one dumbell is held in each hand. A barbell looks similar to a dumbell, but has a much longer bar: you grip the bar with both hands at the same time. Ankle weights are padded strips of fabric that you wear strapped around each ankle: they have pockets in the fabric to hold the weights. When you choose your weight training equipment, remember to buy a type on which the weights are easily adjustable.

1 Alternate arm press
This exercise is for the arms and shoulders.
Stand with your feet hip width apart, dumbells resting on your shoulders (**a**). Straighten your right arm above your head (**b**), return to the starting position, then straighten your left arm above your head (**c**). Return to the starting position and repeat, alternating arms.

2 Squats
This exercise is for the thighs and buttocks.
Stand with your feet shoulder width apart, dumbells resting on your shoulders (**a**). Keeping your back straight and your head up, squat down as far as you can (**b**). Return to the starting position and repeat.

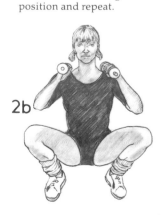

HOW TO EXERCISE

Do not start weight training unless you are already fairly fit. If you are unfit, begin by following a calisthenics programme for a few weeks to build up your muscle strength before beginning your weight training programme. Remember to warm up before and to cool down after your weight training session.

Start training gently using the lightest weights. Begin with 8–10 repetitions of each exercise, and take a short break between each exercise. As you progress, build up to 30 repetitions of each exercise and gradually reduce your rest breaks to a short pause. Once you are comfortable with 30 repetitions, increase the weights by .22–.45kg, and go back to 8–10 repetitions of each exercise. Then build up to 30 repetitions again. Continue to increase the weights in this way until your weights are at a maximum of 2.7kg.

If you decide to make weight training the strength element of your general fitness programme, aim for three 15 minute sessions a week. If you are using weight training to improve or alter your body shape, you will need to aim for 30 minute sessions every 48 hours. Do not exercise with weights every day, or your muscles will not have time to relax. However, if you leave more than 90 hours between sessions your muscles will be too relaxed for you to gain any benefits from the exercises.

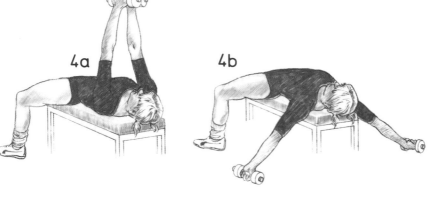

3 Sit up and twist
This exercise is for the waist, hips, and abdomen.
Lie on your back, legs together, holding a dumbell in each hand at shoulder level (**a**). Sit up, bending your knees, and bringing your right elbow forward to touch your left knee (**b**). Return to the starting position and repeat on the other side, bringing your left elbow forward to touch your right knee. Return to the starting position and repeat, alternating sides.

4 Chest flyers
This exercise is for the upper arms and pectoral muscles. Lie on your back on a bench, feet on the floor. Hold your arms straight up above your shoulders with a dumbell in each hand (**a**). Keeping your arms straight, lower the weights downward and out to the sides (**b**). Return to the starting position and repeat.

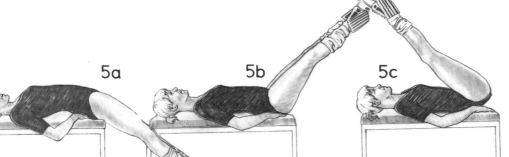

5 Leg raise
This exercise is for the legs, stomach, and hips.
Wear an ankle weight on each leg. Lie on your back on a bench, hands next to your hips, legs together and stretched out in front of you, pointing toward the floor (**a**). Keeping your legs straight, raise them high off the ground (**b**), then bring them back over your body (**c**). Return to the starting position and repeat.

Aerobics

Aerobic simply means "with air." Many different types of exercise – jogging, cycling, and swimming, for example – are aerobic, as they increase your body's need for oxygen. Filling this need makes your heart and lungs work hard, and this hard work makes them fit. Aerobic exercises are therefore the best way of improving your stamina, providing that they are performed steadily and continuously. Exercising strenuously for a few minutes and then resting is not aerobic: to increase your stamina you must keep moving. The exercises that most of us refer to as "aerobics" blend calisthenics and dance movements in a programme that improves your stamina and also makes you stronger and more supple. A good aerobics session will begin with a warm-up, go on to 15–20 minutes of sustained exercise without breaks, and end with cooling down. The exercises are usually performed to rock music, which helps to keep you moving at the right speed and rhythm. You can practise them at home on your own, or go to a class. If you decide on a class, make sure that the teacher has been properly trained. Most of the aerobics injuries that have received so much publicity recently have occurred when untrained teachers have encouraged class members to exercise too hard too soon.

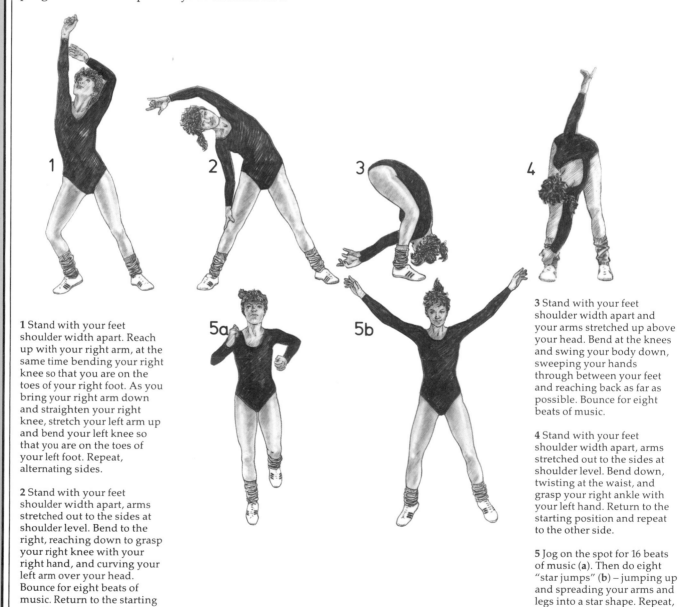

1 Stand with your feet shoulder width apart. Reach up with your right arm, at the same time bending your right knee so that you are on the toes of your right foot. As you bring your right arm down and straighten your right knee, stretch your left arm up and bend your left knee so that you are on the toes of your left foot. Repeat, alternating sides.

2 Stand with your feet shoulder width apart, arms stretched out to the sides at shoulder level. Bend to the right, reaching down to grasp your right knee with your right hand, and curving your left arm over your head. Bounce for eight beats of music. Return to the starting position and repeat to the other side.

3 Stand with your feet shoulder width apart and your arms stretched up above your head. Bend at the knees and swing your body down, sweeping your hands through between your feet and reaching back as far as possible. Bounce for eight beats of music.

4 Stand with your feet shoulder width apart, arms stretched out to the sides at shoulder level. Bend down, twisting at the waist, and grasp your right ankle with your left hand. Return to the starting position and repeat to the other side.

5 Jog on the spot for 16 beats of music (a). Then do eight "star jumps" (b) – jumping up and spreading your arms and legs into a star shape. Repeat, alternating jogging and jumping.

HOW TO EXERCISE

The key to aerobic exercise is your pulse rate. You will get the best results if you exercise hard enough to raise your pulse rate to 70–85% of your maximum safe pulse rate (see p. 41) for 15–20 minutes three times a week. Build up to this level gradually, taking the exercises slowly at first, repeating each one a few times, and resting whenever you need to. As you become fitter, increase the number of repetitions, and the length of your exercise session. Always remember to warm up before and to cool down after your aerobics session. Never "go for the burn": if you feel pain you are exercising too hard and risking muscle damage. Exercising to music will help you keep your movements rhythmic: count the beats out loud if it helps. A wide range of records and tapes of music for aerobics sessions are now available, often with an accompanying chart showing the exercises.

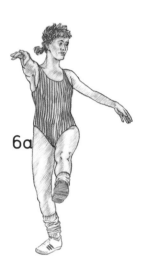

6a

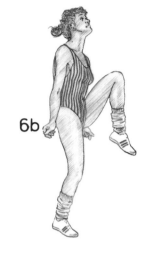

6b

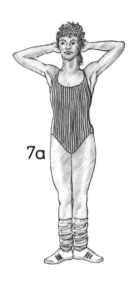

7a

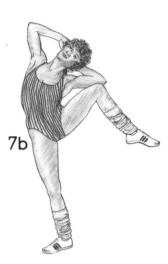

7b

6 Stand with your feet together, arms stretched out to the side at shoulder level. Kick your legs alternately in front of you for 16 beats of music, swinging the opposite arm forward with each leg kick (**a**). Then bring your arms down to your side and hop on alternate feet for 16 beats, bending your free leg and bringing the leg up to your chest on each hop (**b**). Repeat, alternating kicking and jumping.

7 Stand with your feet together and your hands clasped behind your head (**a**). Keep your back straight, head up, and elbows out. Bend sideways, bringing your left knee up to touch your left elbow (**b**). Do not bend forward. Repeat for eight beats of music, then repeat to the other side for eight beats.

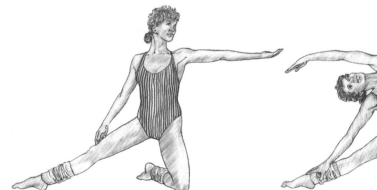

8a

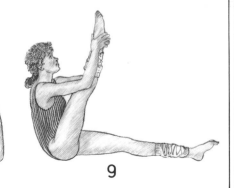

8b

9

8 Kneel on your left knee and stretch your right leg out to the side (**a**). Rest your right hand on your right thigh and stretch your left arm out to the side at shoulder level. Slide your right hand down to your ankle, bringing your left arm up and as far over to the right as possible (**b**). Hold for eight beats of music, then repeat to the other side.

9 Sit on the floor with your legs stretched out in front of you, feet together. Keeping both legs straight, raise your right leg and grasp your right foot and ankle with both hands. Tug your leg toward your face and chest for eight beats of music. Keep your back straight and your head up. Repeat with the other leg.

Walking, jumping, jogging

Jogging, brisk walking (at about 6.4km/h), and jumping rope (skipping) are all excellent aerobic exercises, needing the minimum of equipment. They will help you develop your stamina and strengthen your leg muscles. For all-round fitness you should supplement them with strength exercises for your upper body and a complete programme of suppleness exercises.

WALKING

Because walking is less physically demanding than jogging or other more strenuous forms of aerobic exercise, you need to spend a little more time each week to reach the same level of fitness. Aim to walk briskly for about 45 minutes three times a week. "Briskly" means at a speed of 6.4–8km/h. It is quite easy to check that you are walking at the right speed, 6.4km/h is 120 paces per minute – military marching pace. If you hum a cheerful military march tune as you walk, and keep pace with the beat, you will be walking at approximately the right speed. Build up to this level gently, by walking whenever and wherever you can, and gradually increasing your time and speed.

Make your walking enjoyable by choosing routes that you enjoy – through streets you like, through your local park, or in countryside with good scenery. If you pick a route with plenty of hills you will increase your fitness still farther – walking up a fairly steep hill at 6.4km/h is considered equivalent to running on the flat at 12.8km/h. If you walk in rough country you will probably need specialised walking boots, but otherwise you can walk in any shoes that support your feet comfortably and in which you feel comfortable. Pick flat- or low-heeled shoes: high heels are not really suitable for exercise walking.

A recent trend in exercise walking is known as "power walking". This simply means walking briskly while wearing ankle weights of the type used in weight training. The weights increase the resistance against which your muscles have to work, so helping to make them stronger.

Pulse rate
Remember to check your pulse rate at intervals during these aerobic forms of exercise. Aim to raise your pulse rate to 70–85% of your maximum safe pulse rate (see p. 41) for 15–20 minutes three times a week, but never exercise so hard that you either reach or exceed your maximum safe pulse rate. Remember as well to warm up before and to cool down after your exercise sessions.

JUMPING ROPE

Jumping rope (skipping) for 15 minutes is thought to give you the same amount of exercise as jogging for 30 minutes. The only equipment you need is a rope – either a commercial rope with handles, or a length of sash cord or wash line. Wear shoes that are well cushioned under the balls of your feet to protect your feet and legs from impact damage as you land. Try to jump on a soft surface, such as grass, rather than on concrete, as this will also help to lessen the impact.

Choose any jumping step you like. The simple steps are just as effective for exercise as the fancy jumping steps – although there is nothing to stop you putting in any fancy steps and rope turns that you enjoy. You may also enjoy jumping to music, or playing the jumping and skipping games you played as a child. All you need to remember is to jump lightly (if you can hear yourself land you are jumping too heavily), to keep your knees flexed, and to turn the rope with your wrists, not your hands.

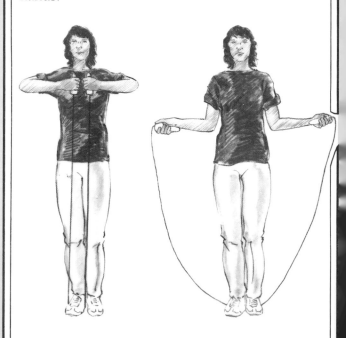

Rope length
To find the correct length of rope for you, stand with one foot on the centre of the rope. The two ends of handles should reach your armpits.

Jumping stance
Stand straight, shoulders relaxed, arms close to your body, forearms out at right angles. Your hands should be at waist level. When you jump, keep your eyes looking straight ahead: don't look at the rope.

JOGGING
How to exercise

If you have never jogged before, start by walking! Make sure that you can walk briskly for at least 15 minutes without feeling any discomfort before you begin to include jogging in your programme. The timetable below shows a possible jogging development programme. If you are very unfit, begin with stage A, then move on to stage B, and so on. If you are reasonably fit to start with, join the programme at any point which feels comfortable and go on from there. Try to exercise every other day during stage A, four times a week during stage B, and five time a week during stage C. When you have completed stage C, maintain your fitness by jogging for about 20 minutes three times a week. Never feel that you have to keep exactly to the times suggested in this programme: progress through it at your own pace.

When you jog, keep your body upright, your back straight, your head up, and your buttocks tucked in. Be relaxed: do not hold your body stiffly. Hold your hands at about waist height, elbows out, forearms parallel to the ground. Keep your hands relaxed: don't clench them into fists. Let your feet strike the ground heel first, then roll forward onto the flat of your foot and push off from your toes. If you try to run on your toes you will get pains in your lower legs. Try to run at an even pace, without lifting your legs high off the ground or pumping hard with your arms. Breathe normally and fairly deeply. If you get out of breath, slow down – if you can't hold a conversation comfortably while you are jogging, you are going too fast!

Shoes

Each of your feet hits the ground approximately 800 times during a one mile jog. If you do not wear proper running shoes, these repeated impacts will damage your feet and legs. Sneakers or shoes intended for other sports are not suitable: buy a proper pair of running shoes before you begin your programme. Get the best pair you can afford and have them fitted by an expert. They should support your feet properly, be well cushioned to minimise impact shock, and flex easily with your feet as you jog. The heel should fit snugly, the shape of the shoe should support the arch of your foot, and there should be enough room for your toes to move easily. When you try on your shoes in the store, wear the socks you intend to wear when you are jogging. Thick cotton socks are probably the most comfortable, and your shoes must fit over them.

	Stage A		Stage B		Stage C	
Week 1	Walk briskly Walk slowly Walk briskly	5 minutes 3 minutes 5 minutes	Walk briskly Walk slowly Walk briskly	10 minutes 3 minutes 10 minutes	Jog Walk Repeat 9 times	40 seconds 1 minute
Week 2	Walk briskly Walk slowly Walk briskly	5 minutes 3 minutes 5 minutes	Walk briskly Walk slowly	15 minutes 3 minutes	Jog Walk Repeat 8 times	1 minute 1 minute
Week 3	Walk briskly Walk slowly Walk briskly	8 minutes 3 minutes 8 minutes	Jog Walk Repeat 12 times	10 seconds 1 minute	Jog Walk Repeat 6 times	2 minutes 1 minute
Week 4	Walk briskly Walk slowly Walk briskly	8 minutes 3 minutes 8 minutes	Jog Walk Repeat 12 times	20 seconds 1 minute	Jog Walk Repeat 4 times	4 minutes 1 minute
Week 5					Jog Walk Repeat 3 times	6 minutes 1 minute
Week 6					Jog Walk Repeat 2 times	8 minutes 2 minutes
Week 7					Jog Walk Repeat 2 times	10 minutes 2 minutes
Week 8					Jog Walk Repeat 2 times	12 minutes 2 minutes

©DIAGRAM

Sports

Taking part in a sport you enjoy can provide all the incentive you need to keep you exercising regularly. But you will need to develop a reasonable level of skill before you can really consider your chosen sport as part of your fitness programme – as an example, you will get very little exercise if you spend most of your tennis matches retrieving the ball from the back of the court!
For most sports, developing the necessary skills will mean going to classes or coaching sessions. These sessions often include training exercises: practised regularly, these exercises will not only help you improve your performance in a sport but will also make you fitter.
Whichever sport you choose, you will get the greatest fitness benefits if you aim for at least three energetic 30 minute sessions each week. The sports described on these pages are particularly useful as part of an exercise programme. Remember that different sports make different demands on your body, and that some will need supplementing with other types of exercise for all-round fitness.

SWIMMING
Swimming helps strengthen muscles, increase suppleness, and improve stamina. The water resists your movements, and it is working against this resistance that makes swimming such a very effective form of exercise. It is particularly useful for anyone who is overweight, or who has back or leg problems – because the water supports your weight it is possible to exercise energetically without risking muscle or joint damage.

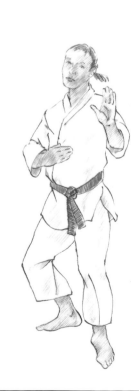

Swimming can only be useful as exercise if you swim vigorously. Aim to complete one length of a 50m pool in about 1½ minutes, and to keep up this rate for 15–20 minutes. Vary strokes for the best results. Front crawl is best for increasing stamina and for improving your body shape; breaststroke strengthens your upper body; backstroke is good for your abdomen, legs, and upper arms; and butterfly exercises your chest, arms, thighs, and shoulders.

MARTIAL ARTS
The oriental martial arts range from the non-combative Tai Chi to the highly aggressive karate. All of them are excellent for developing your suppleness and strength, providing that you have learned them properly from a qualified instructor. The more aggressive martial arts will also help you to develop your stamina, as classes usually include 15–20 minutes of sustained exercises.

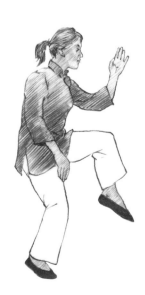

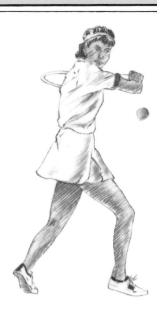

RACKET SPORTS

Squash and racquetball are more physically demanding than tennis and badminton, but any of the racket sports will help you improve your stamina if you play them regularly, energetically, and at a reasonable level of skill. The twisting and turning involved will help you improve your suppleness, but may also put you at risk of damaging your joints and ligaments if you are not fairly flexible already. Watch out too for uneven muscle development – because your racket arm is doing most of the work, it may become stronger than your other arm.

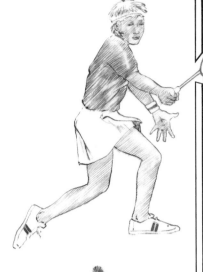

SKIING

There are two main types of skiing – downhill (also called Alpine skiing) and cross-country (also called Nordic skiing or langlauf).
Because downhill skiing alternates short bursts of strenuous activity with rests and rides on ski-lifts, it does not usually provide enough steady, sustained exercise to help you improve your stamina. However, you can use it as a stamina exercise if you can develop enough skill to be able to tackle runs that need 15–20 minutes of continuous skiing. Downhill skiing is very useful for developing strength and suppleness in your legs, especially if you practise pre-ski exercises regularly.
Cross-country skiing is one of the best and most demanding forms of all-round exercise. It exercises nearly all the major muscle groups in your body, and because you can ski continuously for long periods, it is also an excellent stamina exercise.

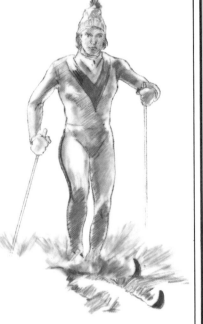

CYCLING

Cycling will help you improve your stamina and strengthen your leg muscles, providing you cycle at a minimum speed of 16–24km/h and keep up this pace for at least 15–20 minutes. For best results, pedal up hills instead of dismounting and walking up, or cycle along the flat using a gear that offers plenty of resistance for your muscles to work against. For all-round fitness, supplement cycling with strength exercises for the upper part of your body and with a full programme of suppleness exercises. Cycling is not recommended for anyone with back problems as the riding position can make them worse.

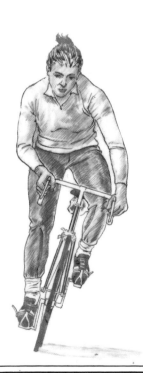

Figure improvement 1

Have you ever wished that you had a flatter, firmer stomach, or tauter buttocks, or trimmer thighs? Practising the exercises shown on these pages can help you to alter the shape of the "problem" areas of your body – providing that you persevere. You will need to exercise every day for at least a month in order to see any results.

These exercises are in addition to your general fitness programme, not a part of it. Some of them are very strenuous, and you should not attempt them unless you are already fairly fit. Pick out the

exercises for the parts of your body that you wish to reshape and work at them daily. You will find that some parts of your body respond more quickly than others. It is relatively easy to flatten your abdomen, but thighs are notoriously slow to change. And because there are no muscles in your breasts, you can only alter the shape of your bust line by exercising the muscles around your breasts and by working to improve your posture. Don't become disheartened – if you keep exercising, your shape will improve.

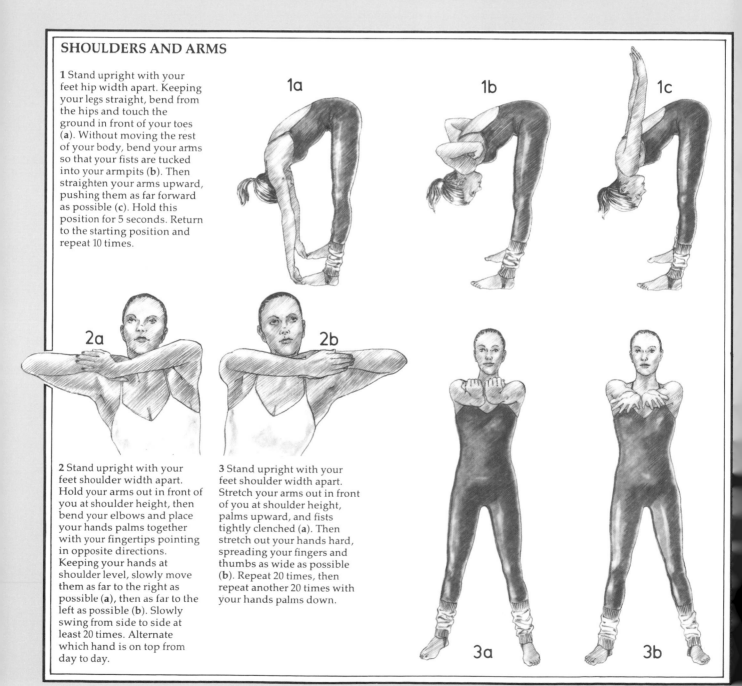

SHOULDERS AND ARMS

1 Stand upright with your feet hip width apart. Keeping your legs straight, bend from the hips and touch the ground in front of your toes (**a**). Without moving the rest of your body, bend your arms so that your fists are tucked into your armpits (**b**). Then straighten your arms upward, pushing them as far forward as possible (**c**). Hold this position for 5 seconds. Return to the starting position and repeat 10 times.

2 Stand upright with your feet shoulder width apart. Hold your arms out in front of you at shoulder height, then bend your elbows and place your hands palms together with your fingertips pointing in opposite directions. Keeping your hands at shoulder level, slowly move them as far to the right as possible (**a**), then as far to the left as possible (**b**). Slowly swing from side to side at least 20 times. Alternate which hand is on top from day to day.

3 Stand upright with your feet shoulder width apart. Stretch your arms out in front of you at shoulder height, palms upward, and fists tightly clenched (**a**). Then stretch out your hands hard, spreading your fingers and thumbs as wide as possible (**b**). Repeat 20 times, then repeat another 20 times with your hands palms down.

BUST AND POSTURE

1 Stand upright or sit cross-legged on the floor. Grasp your hands behind your back as shown in the illustration. Pull up with your top hand and pull down with your lower hand. Keep your body upright: do not bend forward or slump. Hold this position for 5 seconds, then reverse your arm positions and repeat. Repeat 10 times, alternating arm positions.

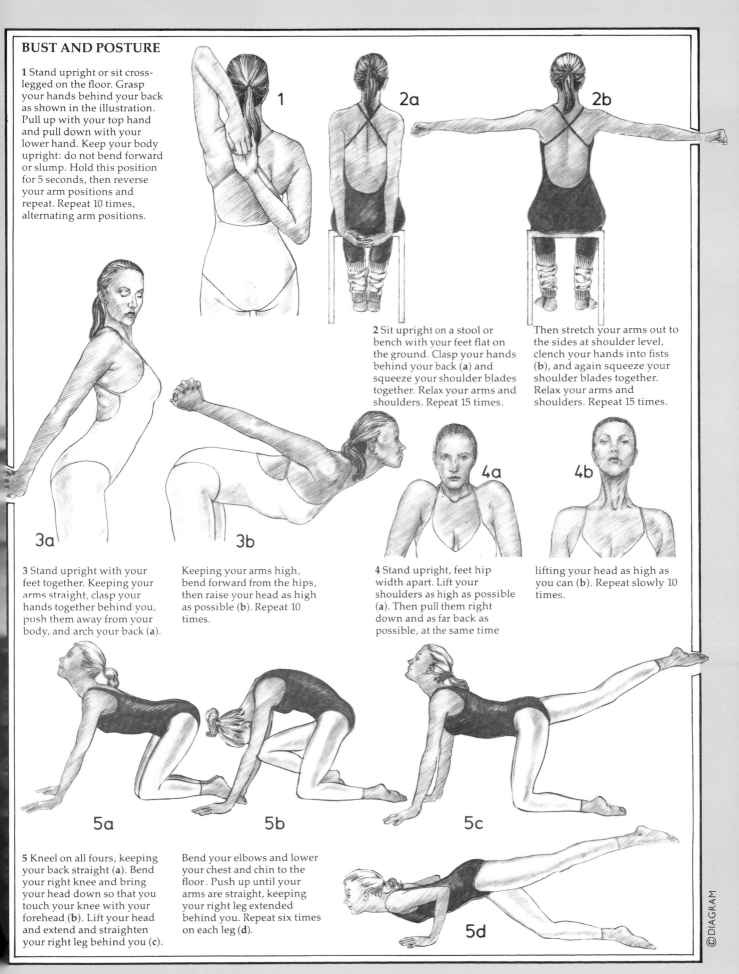

2 Sit upright on a stool or bench with your feet flat on the ground. Clasp your hands behind your back (**a**) and squeeze your shoulder blades together. Relax your arms and shoulders. Repeat 15 times.

Then stretch your arms out to the sides at shoulder level, clench your hands into fists (**b**), and again squeeze your shoulder blades together. Relax your arms and shoulders. Repeat 15 times.

3 Stand upright with your feet together. Keeping your arms straight, clasp your hands together behind you, push them away from your body, and arch your back (**a**).

Keeping your arms high, bend forward from the hips, then raise your head as high as possible (**b**). Repeat 10 times.

4 Stand upright, feet hip width apart. Lift your shoulders as high as possible (**a**). Then pull them right down and as far back as possible, at the same time

lifting your head as high as you can (**b**). Repeat slowly 10 times.

5 Kneel on all fours, keeping your back straight (**a**). Bend your right knee and bring your head down so that you touch your knee with your forehead (**b**). Lift your head and extend and straighten your right leg behind you (**c**).

Bend your elbows and lower your chest and chin to the floor. Push up until your arms are straight, keeping your right leg extended behind you. Repeat six times on each leg (**d**).

©DIAGRAM

Figure improvement 2

HIPS AND BUTTOCKS

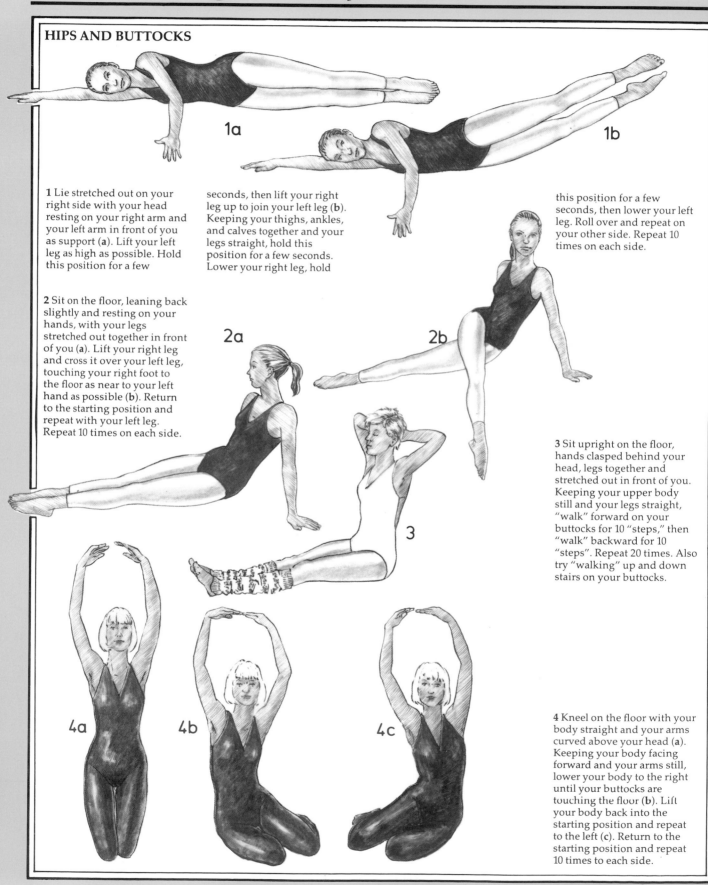

1a

1b

1 Lie stretched out on your right side with your head resting on your right arm and your left arm in front of you as support (**a**). Lift your left leg as high as possible. Hold this position for a few seconds, then lift your right leg up to join your left leg (**b**). Keeping your thighs, ankles, and calves together and your legs straight, hold this position for a few seconds. Lower your right leg, hold this position for a few seconds, then lower your left leg. Roll over and repeat on your other side. Repeat 10 times on each side.

2 Sit on the floor, leaning back slightly and resting on your hands, with your legs stretched out together in front of you (**a**). Lift your right leg and cross it over your left leg, touching your right foot to the floor as near to your left hand as possible (**b**). Return to the starting position and repeat with your left leg. Repeat 10 times on each side.

2a

2b

3

3 Sit upright on the floor, hands clasped behind your head, legs together and stretched out in front of you. Keeping your upper body still and your legs straight, "walk" forward on your buttocks for 10 "steps," then "walk" backward for 10 "steps". Repeat 20 times. Also try "walking" up and down stairs on your buttocks.

4a

4b

4c

4 Kneel on the floor with your body straight and your arms curved above your head (**a**). Keeping your body facing forward and your arms still, lower your body to the right until your buttocks are touching the floor (**b**). Lift your body back into the starting position and repeat to the left (**c**). Return to the starting position and repeat 10 times to each side.

WAIST AND ABDOMEN

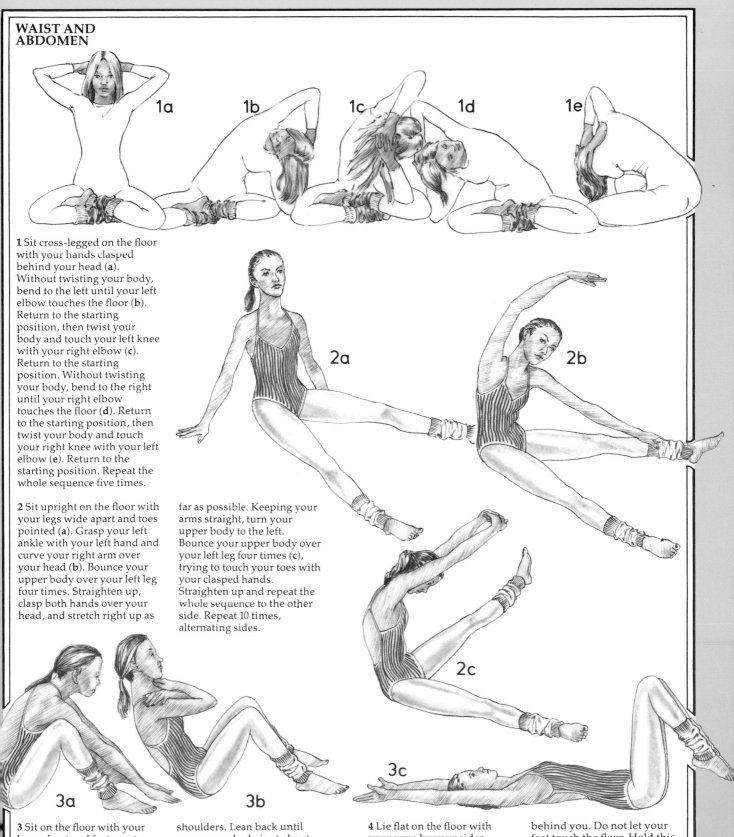

1 Sit cross-legged on the floor with your hands clasped behind your head (**a**). Without twisting your body, bend to the left until your left elbow touches the floor (**b**). Return to the starting position, then twist your body and touch your left knee with your right elbow (**c**). Return to the starting position. Without twisting your body, bend to the right until your right elbow touches the floor (**d**). Return to the starting position, then twist your body and touch your right knee with your left elbow (**e**). Return to the starting position. Repeat the whole sequence five times.

2 Sit upright on the floor with your legs wide apart and toes pointed (**a**). Grasp your left ankle with your left hand and curve your right arm over your head (**b**). Bounce your upper body over your left leg four times. Straighten up, clasp both hands over your head, and stretch right up as far as possible. Keeping your arms straight, turn your upper body to the left. Bounce your upper body over your left leg four times (**c**), trying to touch your toes with your clasped hands. Straighten up and repeat the whole sequence to the other side. Repeat 10 times, alternating sides.

3 Sit on the floor with your knees bent and feet apart. With your arms stretched out together in front of you, bend forward through your knees and touch the floor as far in front of your feet as possible (**a**). Then cross your arms, putting your hands on your shoulders. Lean back until your upper body is at about 45° to the floor (**b**). Hold this position for a few seconds, then bring your body up and forward until your elbows are between your knees. Uncross your arms. Repeat 10 times.

4 Lie flat on the floor with your arms by your sides. Bend your legs and lift your knees up to touch your chest. Keeping your knees bent, lower your feet toward the floor, at the same time lifting your arms up and back so they are touching the floor behind you. Do not let your feet touch the floor. Hold this position for a few seconds. Then lift both knees back to your chest, at the same time bringing your arms up and forward so that they are back by your sides. Repeat 10 times.

Figure improvement 3

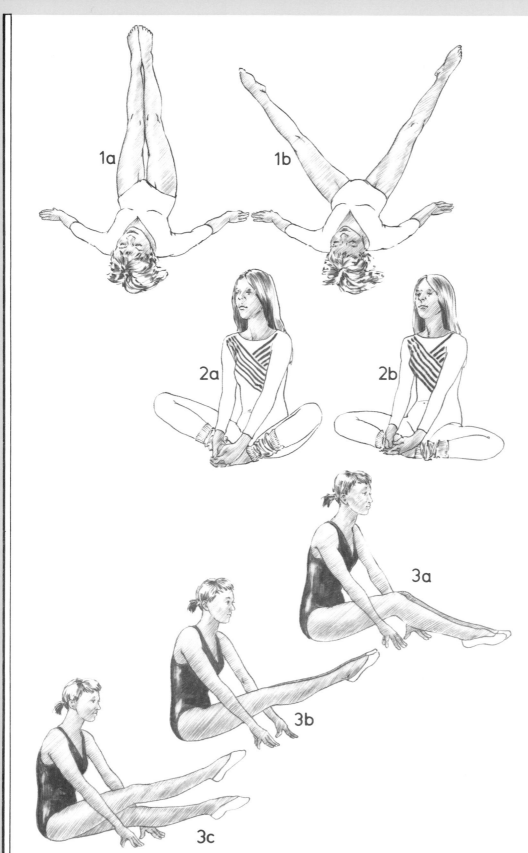

THIGHS AND LEGS

1 Lie on your back with your legs together and raised at right angles to your body, hands by your sides, palms down (**a**). Keeping your legs straight, swing them out to the sides as far as possible (**b**), then return to the starting position. Repeat 20 times.

2 Sit upright on the floor, head up, knees bent, soles of your feet together, and grasp your feet with your hands, keeping your arms straight (**a**). Pull up on your feet and lower your knees outward toward the floor (**b**). Keep your head up and your back straight, and hold this position for 20 seconds. Relax your arms and raise your knees. Repeat five times.

3 Sit on the floor with your lower back against a wall, knees bent, feet on the floor, hands on either side of your knees, fingertips resting on the floor (**a**). Leaning on your fingertips, lift both legs as high off the floor as possible, then straighten your legs and point your toes (**b**). Make scissors movements with your legs, crossing your right leg over your left, then your left foot over your right (**c**). Do 10 scissors movements, then return to the starting position. Repeat 10 times.

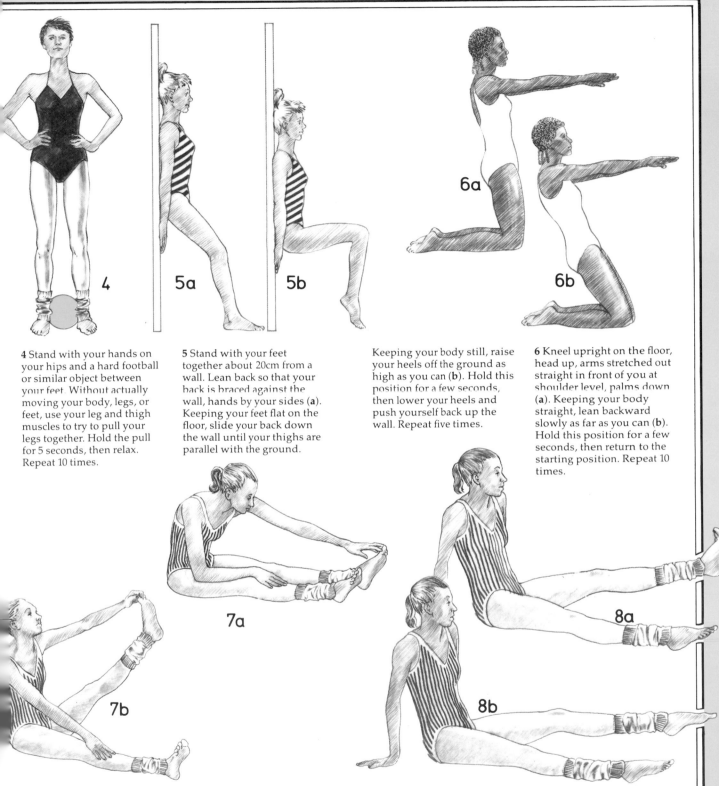

4 Stand with your hands on your hips and a hard football or similar object between your feet. Without actually moving your body, legs, or feet, use your leg and thigh muscles to try to pull your legs together. Hold the pull for 5 seconds, then relax. Repeat 10 times.

5 Stand with your feet together about 20cm from a wall. Lean back so that your back is braced against the wall, hands by your sides (**a**). Keeping your feet flat on the floor, slide your back down the wall until your thighs are parallel with the ground.

Keeping your body still, raise your heels off the ground as high as you can (**b**). Hold this position for a few seconds, then lower your heels and push yourself back up the wall. Repeat five times.

6 Kneel upright on the floor, head up, arms stretched out straight in front of you at shoulder level, palms down (**a**). Keeping your body straight, lean backward slowly as far as you can (**b**). Hold this position for a few seconds, then return to the starting position. Repeat 10 times.

7 Sit on the floor with your legs stretched out in front of you, feet together, then lean forward and grasp your left foot with your left hand (**a**). Keeping your right leg on the floor and your left leg straight, lift your left leg as high as possible (**b**). Keep your left leg in the air, and bend and straighten it five times. Lower your left leg and repeat with your right leg. Repeat five times on each side.

8 Sit on the floor with your legs straight out in front of you, hands on the floor behind you to support your weight. Lift your left leg a few inches off the ground. Keeping your leg straight, pull your toes toward you as hard as possible (**a**), then flex them away from you, stretching your foot and pointing your toes (**b**). Repeat 20 times. Still keeping your left leg in the air, make 20 clockwise circles with your left foot, then 20 counterclockwise circles. Lower your left leg and repeat with your right leg. Repeat the whole exercise twice with each leg.

Chapter 2

your body

Caring for your body means caring for every part of it. Your skin is the largest organ in your body – make sure that yours is always in the peak of condition, whether it is exposed on a beach in the summer sunshine or hidden beneath layers of clothes in the winter cold. You use your hands to express yourself and they attract a great deal of attention – give them the attention they deserve and they will always look lovely. Your feet bear all the strains and stresses of a busy day – make sure that you know how to protect and care for them, or their misery will show in your face.

Personal freshness

Sweat does not smell. The unpleasant body odour we associate with sweat only occurs when the sweat has remained so long on the skin that the body's natural bacteria have been able to make it decompose. These bacteria flourish in warm, damp surroundings – in the areas where sweat is trapped by our clothing, for example, or the parts of our bodies where fresh air does not circulate easily, such as under the arms. Removing sweat from the skin before it has a chance to decompose will prevent odour: for most people this means a daily bath or shower, clean clothes, and an underarm anti-perspirant or deodorant.

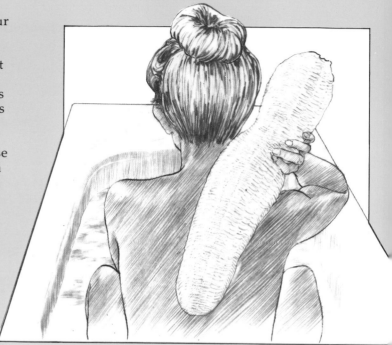

KEEPING FRESH

Wash regularly A daily bath or shower will remove sweat from the skin before it has a chance to decompose. A mild soap and a clean sponge or washcloth are all that you need to keep fresh. Using anti-bacterial or deodorizing soaps, or adding disinfectant to your bathwater, will only destroy your body's essential natural bacteria and protective acid mantle that help to fight invading germs. Remember that your hair needs regular washing for freshness too.

Wear clean clothes Keeping your body clean will not help you keep fresh unless you change and wash your clothes regularly. Sweat clings to clothing, especially to synthetic fabrics, and soon becomes stale and smells unpleasant. Loose fitting clothes in natural fibres allow sweat to evaporate away more easily; close fitting clothes can be protected by purchased dress shields.

Use an anti-perspirant or deodorant regularly These products offer extra protection for the underarm area. If used daily, the level of protection gradually builds up. Always apply anti-perspirants and deodorants to clean, cool, dry skin, and allow them to dry thoroughly before dressing. Deodorant sprays for the feet can also be useful in hot weather. Do not use vaginal deodorants: soap and water are all that are needed to keep the vaginal area clean. The vagina itself is self-cleansing, and deodorant sprays and tissues can upset the delicate balance of its natural secretions and so cause irritations and allergies. The vagina only smells unpleasant if some infection is present. If the odour persists, do not try to mask it with deodorants, but consult your doctor to deal with the underlying cause of the problem.

Watch your diet Poor digestion, heavily spiced food, excessive alcohol, smoking, and poor dental hygiene can all cause bad breath and other unpleasant odours. Taking care of your general health will help you to keep fresh.

BATHS OR SHOWERS?

A warm bath is a lovely way to relax and unwind, but make sure it is warm and not hot. Too hot a bath will make you sweat, can damage your skin (making it age more rapidly), and may cause some of the tiny blood vessels in your body to break. Never remain in a bath so long that your body skin takes on a wrinkled, waterlogged look.

A shower is invigorating, as the pressure of the water helps to speed up your circulation. Like a bath it should be warm and not hot, or it can have the same damaging effects. Showers are probably more useful than baths for getting you fresh as the water pouring over you is clean – while in a bath you are soaking in your own dirt! Combine the two to get the best of both worlds. Either use a shower to rinse away the soap and scum after your bath, or wash first under the shower and then enjoy a relaxing soak in clean bath water.

ANTI-PERSPIRANTS AND DEODORANTS

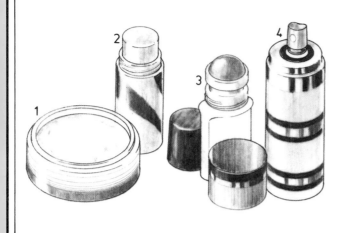

Anti-perspirants contain aluminum salts that act as an astringent. When these salts come into contact with the skin they dehydrate the sweat glands so that sweat production is reduced by as much as 50%. Most anti-perspirants also contain a deodorant, but deodorants on their own do not reduce the amount of sweat produced. They consist of a perfume, intended to disguise any odour produced, and an anti-bacterial agent to slow down the sweat/bacteria reaction. Anti-perspirants and deodorants are available as creams (**1**), sticks (**2**), roll-ons (**3**), and aerosols (**4**). Creams tend to have the strongest formulation; sticks and roll-ons are usually more effective than aerosols. Because the formulae vary so much from brand to brand, experiment to find the best product for you. Once you find the variety that suits you, stay with it: there is no evidence to suggest that repeated use of a particular brand makes it less effective. Do change your brand if it causes you any type of allergic reaction. Unperfumed products are less likely to cause these reactions than the perfumed varieties, and have the added advantage of not clashing with your chosen scent.

WASHING EQUIPMENT

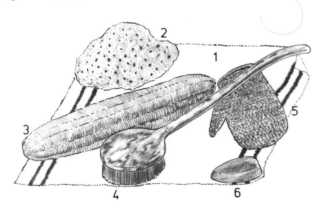

1 Washcloth
It is very important to keep your washcloth clean and to replace it regularly, or it will become an excellent breeding ground for bacteria. Rinse it thoroughly every time you use it. Boil it at least once a week, adding a tablespoon of lemon juice or vinegar to the water to remove soap slime.

2 Sponge
Natural sea sponges are expensive and deserve care. Rinse your sponge thoroughly in clean water every time you use it, and leave it to dry somewhere where all the water can drain away from it. A sponge that is left to stand in water will soon rot.

3 Loofah
A loofah is actually a dried vegetable gourd. When you buy one it is flat: soak it in hot water and it will swell up. Its rough surface helps to remove dead skin cells and keep your skin soft and smooth. Rinse and drain loofahs as for natural sponges, or they will go black and moldy.

4 Back brush
Unless you have someone handy to scrub your back for you, you will need a back brush or friction strap to get your back clean. Pick one with an abrasive action that will remove dead skin: this will help to prevent blackheads and spots developing on your back.

5 Friction mitt
This is an alternative to a loofah for removing dead skin cells, smoothing rough skin, and stimulating circulation. A mitt is most effective if you use it before your bath or shower: if this feels too harsh on your skin, use it when you are actually in the water.

6 Pumice stone
This is a piece of porous volcanic rock that provides a firm abrasive for removing rough or hard skin from your feet or elbows. Synthetic pumice stones are also available. Work up a good soapy lather and then rub the stone on your skin with brisk circular movements.

SWEAT PRODUCTION

There are two types of sweat glands in the body – the eccrine glands and the apocrine glands. The eccrine glands are found all over the body (**1**) and are part of the body's temperature control system: the evaporation of the sweat from these glands cools the body when it becomes too hot. Sweat from the eccrine glands is 99% water and 1% sodium chloride (salt).

The apocrine glands are found associated with areas of body hair (**2**) – under the arms, in the pubic area, and around the nipples. They produce sweat in response to nervous or emotional changes in your body. Sweat from the apocrine glands contains pheromones – chemicals that are said to act as a signal to the opposite sex.

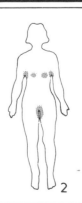

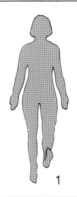

© DIAGRAM

Special baths

Make the most of your bath by using it for beauty treatments as well as for getting yourself clean and fresh. The steam from a warm bath will help a face or hair pack to work well, or will soften your nails and cuticles ready for a manicure or pedicure. Bath additives can be used to improve your skin, or to relax or invigorate you – or simply to make you feel glamorous as you soak surrounded by a froth of bubbles.

COMMERCIAL BATH ADDITIVES

Bath salts and crystals These are made from sodium carbonate (washing soda) and soften the water as well as scenting and colouring it. They are very useful if you live in a hard water area.

Bubble baths These are made from detergent with a stabiliser added to prevent the foam disappearing too quickly. Avoid them if you have dry skin, as they remove the skin's natural oils.

Bath gels Unlike other bath additives, these are intended to clean your skin as you soak. They are mild enough to suit most skins.

Bath milks Like bath salts, these are basically water softeners. Some brands contain moisturisers to help dry skins. Avoid them if you have an oily skin, as they will make it worse.

Bath oils These protect dry skins from the effects of the water, and are designed to moisturise your skin. They are not suitable for anyone with an oily skin. Two types are available: floating oils, which remain on the surface of the water and cling to your skin as you get out of the bath, and emulsifying oils, which disperse through the water. Bath oils can also be rubbed into your skin before you get into the bath.

Bath essences These simply scent the water, and are often available to match your favourite perfume. Choose an alcohol-based essence if you have an oily skin, and an oil-based essence if you have dry skin.

ALTERNATIVE BATHS

The less you wear in these baths, the more effective they are! Always remove your watch and all your jewellery, as they will become hot and may burn you. Wrap a towel around your head to protect your hair.

Saunas

In a traditional suana you lie on a bench in a wood-lined room, heated by a stove on the top of which are several large stones. Ladling water onto these stones produces bursts of steam which ionize the otherwise dry air in the sauna.

Sauna temperatures vary from 150–230°F (65–110°C): the higher benches are hotter than the lower benches. The heat raises your temperature, dilates your blood vessels, makes you sweat, increases your circulation, and draws impurities from your skin.

Do not remain in a sauna for too long: alternate spells of 10–20 minutes with a cold shower or a plunge in a cold pool. Saunas are only for the healthy: avoid them if you have heart trouble, blood pressure problems, respiratory or circulation problems, or if you have recently had surgery or a major illness. They are also inadvisable for pregnant women.

Because saunas reduce the level of fluid in your body you may appear to lose a few pounds in weight during your sauna. However, you will replace this weight as soon as you drink a glass of water and bring your fluid level back to normal. Do not have a meal or drink alcohol within an hour of having a sauna.

Turkish baths

In these baths you move from room to room, each at a different temperature. You usually begin in a dry warm room, move on to a hotter dry room, and them move on to the steam rooms, again working up from warm to hot. After your steam treatment, you will be given a body scrub and massage. A plunge in a cold pool or a cold shower will close your pores again. The watchpoints for Turkish baths are the same as for saunas.

Steam cabinets

These are like a miniature Turkish bath, and because they need so much less room, they are much more easily available. Your body is enclosed in a cabinet, but your head remains outside, well away from the steam. The temperature and amount of steam can be adjusted by the operator, and a towel is wrapped around your neck to prevent the steam escaping. Watchpoints for steam cabinets are the same as for saunas and Turkish baths.

SPECIAL BATHS

Soothing or stimulating baths can easily be prepared from herbs and other household ingredients. Tie herbs, oatmeal, and other solids into a muslin bag: hang it from the taps so that the water flows through it, or simply leave the bag in the bath. Liquids can be added direct to the water and mixed in.

Milk bath Add one pint of milk (or one cup of powdered milk), a spoonful of clear honey, and a little almond oil to the water for a moisturising soothing bath for dry skins.

Vinegar bath Add one cup of cider vinegar to your bath to soften the water and soothe dry or sensitive skin.

Herb and oatmeal bath Mix your choice of herbs with a handful of oatmeal (the oatmeal will soften the bathwater) for a variety of effects. Mint is refreshing and reviving; thyme softens the skin; rosemary stimulates the circulation; camomile opens the pores; and comfrey is good for spotty skin.

Sea salt bath Use two cups of sea salt in your bath to help to draw any impurities from your skin. This bath is particularly good for oily skins. Add some powdered kelp or seaweed (from health stores) as well, and your bath will also help to reduce muscular aches, pains, and tensions.

BODY SCRUBS

The bath is the ideal place to retexturise your skin and to remove any roughness or small lumps and bumps. Friction mitts or body scrubs will keep your skin soft and step up your circulation. Rub them over damp skin as you stand in the bath, using a circular motion and always working toward your heart. Commercial body scrubs are available, or you can make your own. Try handfuls of coarse-grained sea salt or coarse oatmeal; sea salt or sugar mixed to a paste with a bland vegetable oil; or ground almonds mixed with yogurt. Wash off all traces of the scrub in your bath or shower. For a really silky skin, finish off by smoothing in a body lotion as soon as you have dried yourself and while your skin is still warm.

Wax baths

A paraffin wax treatment or wax bath is used to remove dead skin cells, soften the skin, draw off excess body fluids, and act as a muscle relaxant. It can be used all over your body, or simply on a specific part, such as your legs. Cream is smoothed over the part of the body to be treated, and then warm, melted paraffin wax is applied with a brush. Wrapping with foil helps to keep in the heat. The cooled wax is peeled off after about 20 minutes.

Water pressure treatments

Jacuzzis, whirlpool baths, and needle baths all use water under pressure to massage muscles and soft body tissues and stimulate circulation. Jacuzzis and whirlpool baths contain jets around the sides that swirl strong pulses of water around your body. Needle baths have much finer jets that shoot powerful narrow jets of water at you: the temperature is controlled so that warm and cold jets alternate, so dilating and contracting your blood vessels.

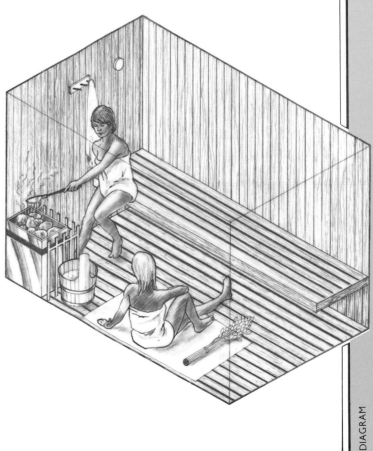

Perfume

The same fragrance – even when taken from the same bottle – will never smell exactly the same on any two women. How a fragrance smells on you depends on your individual body chemistry: your body warmth, the acidity of your skin, and so on all have their effect on the complex mixture of essences in the perfume's formula. Because fragrance is so personal, it is worth spending a little time to choose a perfume that really suits you.

CHOOSING A PERFUME

You will first need to decide on the type of fragrance you want. Are you looking for one that is light and flowery, modern and sophisticated, warm and sensual, or rich and oriental in character? Perfumier's advertisements and the packaging they choose for their fragrances will give you some idea of the character of the scent – you would not expect to find a true flower scent packaged in an oriental style lacquer bottle, for example.

The next step is to try the perfumes that interest you on your skin. Never try more than three or four fragrances on the same day, or your sense of smell will become thoroughly confused. Keep the perfumes well apart on your skin, too, or you will be unable to distinguish one from another – try a sample on the inside of each wrist, and in the crook of each elbow. Wear your test fragrances for at least an hour before making any decision: it takes at least 30 minutes and often longer for the full, true scent to develop on your skin.

Once you have picked a fragrance that you find appealing on your skin, take it away and try it for a few days. This will give you a better chance to see if you really like it, to get your friends' opinions, and to see how other people react. If no samples are available, buy the smallest, cheapest bottle of the fragrance that you can, and try it out in the same way. Perfume is expensive – so any mistakes you make with it are also expensive!

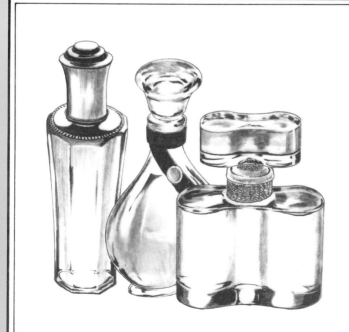

PERFUME STRENGTHS

Extrait or perfume
This consists of 15–20% pure perfume and 80–85% spirit or alcohol, and will last for up to 6 hours on your skin, depending on your body chemistry. It is the most expensive form of perfume, but it is also the strongest and the truest in fragrance.

Parfum de toilette
This is made up of 12–15% pure perfume, up to 85% spirit, and a little water. It is more economical than an extrait or parfum, but longer lasting than eau de toilette. You can expect it to last on your skin for up to 5 hours.

Eau de toilette
This consists of up to 12% pure perfume and a mixture of spirit and water, with a higher proportion of water than spirit. It is lighter than a parfum or parfum de toilette, and so can be used more lavishly. Depending on the amount of water in the formula, it will last for 2–4 hours on your skin.

Eau de cologne
This consists of up to 6% pure perfume, up to 95% water, and a little spirit. It is the lightest form of a fragrance, and will last for only 1–2 hours on your skin.

WEARING PERFUME

The true smell of a fragrance develops best on your pulse points, where your blood vessels are close to the surface of your body and your skin temperature is slightly higher. These points are found on the insides of your wrists, the crooks of your elbows and knees, behind your ears, on the nape of your neck, at the base of your throat, around your ankles, and between your breasts. It is also a good idea to put on your perfume immediately after your bath or shower, while your skin is still warm. But be careful where you apply your perfume if your skin is going to be exposed to the sun. Some perfume formulae contain ingredients that react with your skin in sunlight, leaving a dark stain.

Choose the strength of your fragrance to match the time of day and your choice of activities. Most people prefer the lighter forms of fragrance during the day or when they are at work, building up to the full strength perfumes later in the day or on social occasions. Remember that you will need to reapply your perfume at intervals during the day – how often will depend on the strength of fragrance you are using and your body chemistry.

Many fragrances are now available in a range of products, and you may be able to buy dusting powder, bath oil, and so on to match your perfume. Using these will help to intensify the effect of your chosen fragrance. As an alternative, you could use unscented bath products which would not clash with your perfume. If you mix bath products and perfumes from different ranges, make sure that they are of the same type (all florals, or all citrus, for example), or the combination of fragrances may be less than pleasant. Watch out too for highly scented deodorants and hairsprays, as these may also combine unhappily with your perfume.

Try to avoid getting perfume on your clothes or jewellery, as it can stain or damage them. However, an empty perfume bottle placed in a drawer or closet will add fragrance to your clothes as the last few drops clinging to the inside of the bottle evaporate away.

STORING PERFUME

Exposure to air, light, heat, and moisture makes perfume deteriorate, darken, and lose its character and true smell. Keep your perfume in a cool, dark place and always make sure that the bottle is properly closed. Perfumes in sealed atomisers will last longer than those in bottles – besides being protected from the air, they are also protected from your skin's chemicals and oils. These are transferred to the bottle every time you rub the stopper on your skin or use your fingers to apply your perfume, and they can also cause perfume to deteriorate. Although large bottles of perfume are very glamorous, you will get the best from your fragrance if you only buy bottles that contain enough scent to last you for 6–8 weeks. Remember that the more concentrated the fragrance, the more rapidly it will break down. Keep your fragrance in its original bottle if at all possible. If you must decant it into another container, choose one that is made of glass, not plastic, and make sure that it is perfectly clean and dry with no trace of detergent remaining in it.

PERFUME NOTES

Great perfumiers are noted for their "nose" or perfect sense of smell. They use their skill to blend natural and synthetic oils, essences, and fixatives to produce a particular fragrance. Perfumiers design scents to have three "notes" – three distinct but coordinated levels of fragrance that gradually develop as the perfume remains on your skin.

The top note is the fragrance that you notice as soon as you apply your perfume. It lasts for only 10–20 minutes before giving way to the middle note. The middle note provides the fragrance for 20–30 minutes after the top note has disappeared, so giving the base note plenty of time to develop. The base note is the strongest and longest lasting part of the perfume. Initially it can smell unpleasant on the skin, but this smell is hidden by the top and middle notes. It needs at least 30 minutes for the base note to develop its true fragrance, and it will then last for about 6 hours. Because the base note is the most lasting part of the perfume, it is the perfumier's starting point when a new perfume is being developed. A little residual fragrance is left when the base note has evaporated: this residue is known as the dry-out, and in some circumstances it can last for months, or even years!

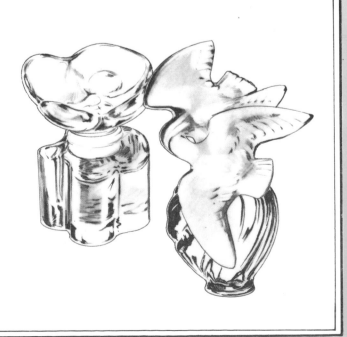

Hair removal

Unwanted hair can be a problem for many women. Hair grows naturally all over the body except on the palms of the hands and soles of the feet. Many women choose to remove hair routinely from underarms and lower legs. Smooth armpits and legs, however, are no longer considered a fashion necessity and many women do not defuzz at all.

More difficult than the routine removal of normal hair growth is the question of dark hair growing coarsely or thickly in certain parts of the body such as around the nipples, or on the face, lower abdomen, or tops of thighs. Unwanted hair in these areas can cause considerable embarrassment but there are several methods you can use to disguise or remove it.

Different methods are suitable for different areas. Shaving the upper lip or forearm, for instance, would be disastrous, leading to coarse, dark stubble which would be impossible to conceal; bleaching the hair in these areas disguises it sufficiently and presents no regrowth problems. Some methods, such as shaving, are short term and need to be repeated frequently. Others, such as waxing, give a longer lasting result. Electrolysis is the only method of hair removal that can claim to be permanent.

Methods of hair removal
Different methods of hair removal are suitable for different parts of the body. Shown below are methods suggested for certain areas.

1 Plucking
2 Bleaching
3 Electrolysis
4 Abrasion
5 Shaving
6 Chemical depilatories
7 Waxing

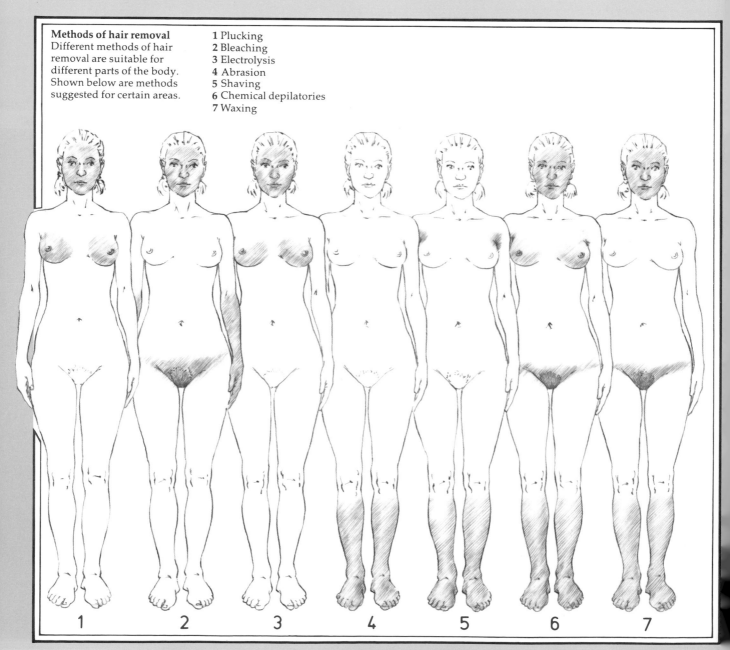

1 2 3 4 5 6 7

Plucking

Plucking is the easiest and safest way to remove a stray hair from your face, breast, or abdomen. Using eyebrow tweezers, you pluck out the hair by its root. The hair grows again but it will not be coarser or thicker. Astringent may be applied before plucking to reduce discomfort. Never pluck a hair from a mole or wart.

Shaving

Shaving is a simple, cheap, and efficient way of removing leg and underarm hair. Because the hair has been cut, however, its blunt end can feel coarse and bristly so you need to shave very regularly to keep your skin soft and smooth. If you use a safety razor, make sure the blade is sharp, and use plenty of baby oil to avoid cutting the skin. Moisturise afterwards.

Waxing

Waxing is a very satisfactory method of hair removal for the legs and bikini line (i.e. the lower abdomen and upper thighs). Regrowth does not appear for several weeks. Usually carried out in a salon, waxing can be done very successfully at home with a little practice. Heated wax is applied to the legs and ripped off as it is on the point of setting. It is less painful than it sounds!

1 Melted wax is applied with a brush.
2 The wax is left to cool.
3 The wax is stripped off the leg, removing the hairs with it.

Bleaching

Bleaching is an excellent way of disguising hair on your arms, legs, and face. A commercial bleaching preparation is applied to the area for the required time, and then rinsed away with clear water. This method is both painless and harmless, though it is important to try a test patch first.

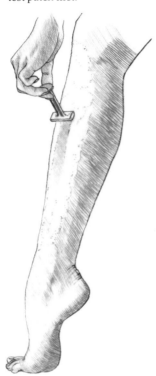

Electrolysis

Electrolysis is the only method of hair removal that can hope to achieve permanent results. A fine needle is inserted into the hair follicle and a tiny electrical current passed down to the root to kill it. If the root is not killed then regrowth occurs. Electrolysis has to be performed by a professional and can be time consuming and expensive. It is, however, the best solution for small areas of hair on the upper lip and chin.

Depilation

Depilation is the term used for the dissolving of unwanted hair by chemicals. Depilatory products are available as creams, gels, powders, or sprays and are applied using a spatula. The substance is then washed away, taking all the hairs with it. The result is quite long lasting and the skin seems smooth. Depilatory products can be used on all sorts of body hair, but carry out a test patch first.

Abrasion

Abrasive pads can be used on your legs to keep hair growth to a minimum. Each pad consists of fine sandpaper and you rub with circular movements to remove the hair. This method is only suitable for the legs where hair growth is quite fine and the skin quite tough. Do not try this method if you have a sensitive skin.

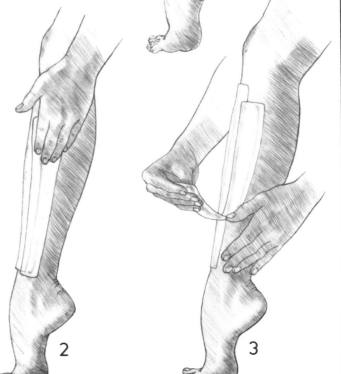

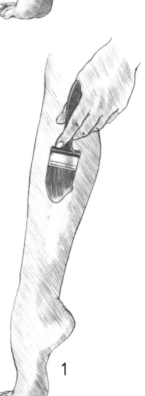

1

2

3

Sun and skin

A healthy looking tan is undoubtedly a great beauty asset and, with the development of fake tans and the availability of sunlamp treatments, one that is no longer confined to those who can afford long holidays on sunny beaches.

But nothing beats a natural tan, achieved by spending time in the sunshine. Sun is a natural source of vitamin D; it has a mildly antiseptic effect which helps fight some skin bacteria; and it has a therapeutic effect on skin affected by acne. Despite its obviously beneficial effects, the sun can also be extremely harmful to your skin. Exposure to too much sunshine causes the skin to dry out, to coarsen, and to lose some of its elasticity. In very rare cases, too much sunshine can lead to forms of skin cancer.

HOW SKIN TANS

Your skin contains a pigment called melanin that gives it its colour. When exposed to the ultraviolet rays of the sun, the skin's natural response is to produce more melanin to protect itself. In this way a tan develops. How quickly and easily you tan depends on your natural melanin concentration and on your body's response to sunshine.

PROTECTING YOUR SKIN

All skin needs protection from prolonged exposure to hot sun and this is especially important if you are fair skinned (i.e. have little natural melanin). Suncare products come in a variety of forms – creams, milks, lotions, and oils – and contain chemicals that help screen out the harmful ultraviolet rays. Many brands carry a protection factor or sunscreen index. The higher protection factor products are for skin that burns easily, and the lower factor products are suitable for skin that has already been exposed to the sun. Sunblocks block out all the ultraviolet rays and are suitable for skins that need total protection.

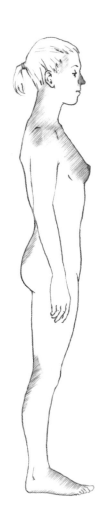

Tanning without burning

Tan gradually. Start with a short session – 10 to 30 minutes depending on skin colour – and build up gradually to longer sessions.

Apply sunscreen before setting off for the beach. Reapply after bathing. Do not forget that a fake tan does not protect you from the real sun – you still need a sunscreen.

Avoid the midday sun.

Protect the most sensitive areas (shown above) with a higher protection factor product if necessary.

Always use an after-sun moisturiser.

If you are burned, apply calamine lotion and keep out of the sun.

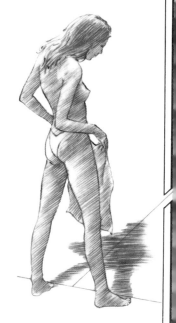

Sun check

Use this simple check to find out if you are risking burning rather than browning as you lie in the sun. Lie down flat, and mark the places where your head and feet touch the ground. Stand on one of these marks so that your shadow points at the other mark – almost as if you were a human sundial. If your shadow is less than your height (i.e. if it falls short of the second mark), be extremely careful how you sunbathe, as the sun is especially burning.

Sun beds and sun lamps

Sun bed and sun lamp treatments simulate the sun's natural ultraviolet rays and help you achieve an attractive, natural looking tan. Treatments help in stimulating the body's natural defence mechanism and therefore can be a helpful prelude to a holiday in the sun.

Time yourself carefully. You can burn as easily as you can in natural sunshine. Aim to build up your tan gradually over several sessions.

Always wear goggles to protect your eyes.

If you are taking any drugs, check with a doctor before embarking on tanning sessions as an allergic reaction can result.

Sun beds utilise tubes which produce ultraviolet A rays which do not tend to severely burn, but are acknowledged by dermatologists to penetrate deep through the epidermis and affect the collagen/ elastin structures. Therefore, extreme care should be exercised in order to avoid long term aging effects to the skin.

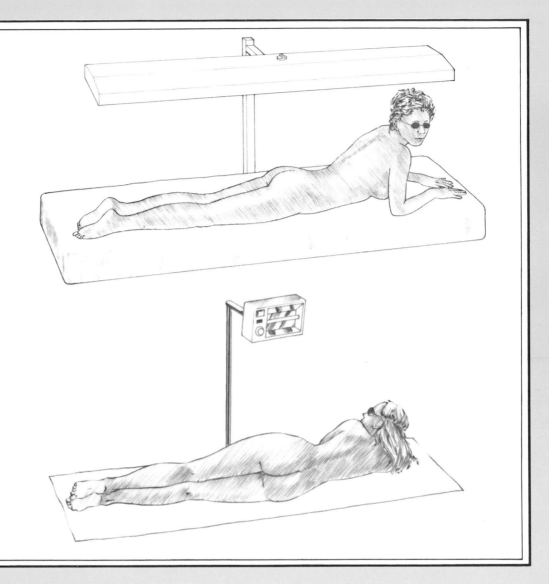

FAKE TANS

If you want a tan and cannot spend time in the sun, then you can try one of the many excellent artificial tanning products now available. You can choose between an instant tint which colours the skin immediately and can be washed off with soap and water, or a colour developing cream which takes up to six hours to mature and which fades naturally.

Instant tints are available in three forms – lotions, creams, and gels. Lotions should be applied on cotton pads to give a good, even coverage. They are spirit-based, so as the alcohol evaporates, the colour remains to stain the skin. Several applications may be needed for a deep golden tan. Tinted creams and gels are also applied using cotton pads or a sponge. They can be more difficult to manage than lotions, so beware of streaking. Products in this form tend to be bright orange; the colour mellows as it is applied. Take care to blend in the creams and gels thoroughly or you may find a tell-tale line where your tan finishes!

Colour developing creams need very careful application. They are white in colour and it is impossible to see whether you are applying them evenly. Several very light coats are better than one heavy one. Use the creams sparingly on areas of hard skin as the dye is absorbed more readily in these areas, and if you are not careful, you will end up with unsightly dark brown or orange patches. To achieve the best possible results from any fake tan, remember the following hints.

Moisturise your skin thoroughly first to ensure even coverage.

Apply the product thinly, swiftly, and as evenly as you can.

Use several light applications rather than one heavy one. Be particularly wary of knees, elbows, and heels which may need only one coat.

Ask a friend to help you reach parts which you cannot see very well – especially your back.

Wash your hands immediately you have finished, or your palms will be stained brown or orange.

©DIAGRAM

Skin problems

The skin on your body deserves as much care as the skin on your face. Good diet, plenty of exercise, enough sleep, and so on will help to keep it in peak condition. Many of the skin problems that may affect your face can also affect your body, and can be treated in the same way (see pp. 110–111); others are described here.

Stretch marks
These may appear as a result of pregnancy or because of major fluctuations in weight. They are caused when the lower layers of the skin are stretched so much that they tear, leaving long white or transparent-looking scars. Stretch marks are usually found on the breasts, abdomen, hips, and thighs. Once you have them, they are permanent (unless you decide on cosmetic surgery), but they do fade to very fine silvery lines in time.

To some extent, whether you will develop stretch marks or not is genetically determined. You are less likely to develop them if you keep fit and healthy, avoid becoming overweight, and moisturise your skin regularly so that it remains supple. During pregnancy, you should eat foods that are high in zinc and vitamin C, as these are thought to be helpful in preventing stretch marks. Because the tears and scarring occur in the deeper levels of the dermis, massaging the skin during pregnancy with special creams is not particularly useful.

Cellulite
Experts disagree as to whether cellulite exists. The term is usually used to refer to the dimpled fat deposits often found on the hips, buttocks, thighs, and upper arms. The skin in these areas takes on a crinkled, pitted appearance, looking rather like orange peel.

Whether these deposits are cellulite or simply ordinary fat, they are very difficult to move, but good diet, exercise, drinking plenty of water, and massage will all help. The wide range of treatments, creams, and so on claimed to remove cellulite are rarely of any use.

Allergies
If you develop a sudden rash, itching, or reddening of the skin, you may have an allergy. Perfumes and chemicals in bath products and deodorants are a common cause of allergies, and the simple cure is to stop using the product that causes the problem. If you have a sensitive skin, try using unscented or hypo-allergenic products. Allergies can of course have other causes – you may be allergic to something you have eaten, something you are wearing, or to a piece of jewellery. You may be able to eliminate the source of the problem by trial and error. If the allergy persists, consult your doctor, who may be able to offer you desensitising treatment.

Poor skin colour
Pale or sallow skins can be improved by stepping up your circulation using exercise, friction mitts, massage, and so on. If your skin occasionally becomes blotchy, it is probably an emotional reaction to stress; if the blotchiness is more persistent, it is again probably caused by poor circulation.

MEDICAL CONDITIONS
Some skin conditions require professional medical treatment and you should consult your doctor if you suspect that you suffer from any of the following.

Hives This is also known as urticaria or nettle rash. Itchy, raised, reddish weals surrounded by white rings may appear anywhere on the body.
Dermatitis This is an allergic reaction which makes the skin burn, itch, or sting, and often produces a rash which may ooze clear fluid.

Eczema This is marked by red, raised patches on the skin, groups of skin eruptions or blisters, and chronic itching. It often first develops in infancy.
Psoriasis This is a chronic but non-contagious condition in which the skin develops bright red patches covered by silvery scales.
Fungal infections The most common of these is ringworm, which produces expanding, itchy, scaly rings on the body.

MARKS ON THE SKIN

Brown spots Also known as liver spots, these may appear as you get older. They can be treated with special fading or bleaching creams, or hidden by camouflage make-up.

Thread veins Also known as red veins or spider veins, these often appear on the legs. They are caused when small blood vessels near the surface of the skin get broken. These breakages can be caused by excessive heat or cold, high blood pressure, or injuries. Professional treatment is required to remove them, using either sclerotherapy (which uses an electric needle and special chemicals to drain the blood vessels) or laser therapy.

Scorch marks These red marks on the legs are actually mild burns, usually caused by sitting too close to a fire. They can take several months to fade, so make sure that you protect your legs from excessive heat.

Vitilgo In this skin condition, small areas of the skin remain white, looking rather like white freckles. Exposure to the sun can make the condition worse. Treatment with drugs may be available from your doctor, or you can camouflage the marks with cosmetics.

Chloasma These dark, coin-shaped patches on the skin are caused by an inherited tendency to react to the female sex hormones, either during pregnancy or when taking the contraceptive pill. Exposure to the sun can make the patches darker. They will usually fade with time when hormone levels have been reduced to normal.

Linea nigra This is a brown line running downward from the navel which may develop in pregnant women. The whole of the abdominal skin may also become darker in pregnancy. The line and the colour both usually fade when the child is born.

BODY WATCHPOINTS

Neck The skin on your neck is often the first to suffer as you get older. It can develop a crepey appearance, losing its elasticity and becoming marked with criss-cross lines. Remember to cleanse your neck thoroughly to prevent it becoming dingy, especially in winter when it is well wrapped up in high-necked sweaters or scarves. Massage in plenty of moisturiser, using gentle upward strokes. You may want to use a richer moisturiser than you use on your face, or perhaps a special throat cream.

Back and shoulders Pay particular attention to these areas if you have an oily skin or a tendency to get blackheads or spots. Sweat and oil trapped by your clothes can sometimes make these problems worse on your back than on your face – and because you cannot see your back, it is only too easy to forget about it!

Elbows Most of us rest on our elbows several times a day. Because of this, the skin on our elbows can become rough and discoloured. Body scrubs, friction mitts, or pumice stones can all be used to make elbows smoother. Discolouration can be dealt with by resting each elbow in half a squeezed lemon for about 15 minutes – the lemon juice remaining in the skins will act as a bleaching agent. You could also try applying a face pack to your elbows: the brush on/peel off type are particularly useful for removing dead skin cells.

Knees Knees can suffer from the same problems as elbows, and merit similar treatment with body scrubs, lemon skin rubs, and so on.

Shins Most of the skin on your body is protected from the weather by your clothes – but legs are often exposed to extremes of hot and cold. Use plenty of moisturiser on the skin of your shins to protect them from becoming dry and flaky.

SKIN STRUCTURE

The top layer of the skin, the epidermis, is made up of dead skin cells that form a tough, flexible, waterproof barrier that keeps harmful substances outside the body. Below the epidermis is a thicker layer called the dermis. The dense and elastic dermis contains the sebaceous glands (which secrete the body's natural oils), sweat glands, hair follicles, nerve endings, blood vessels, and so on. A cushioning layer of subcutaneous tissue (fat) lies underneath the dermis.

a Epidermis
b Dermis
c Subcutaneous tissue
d Sebaceous gland
e Nerve
f Hair follicle
g Sweat gland

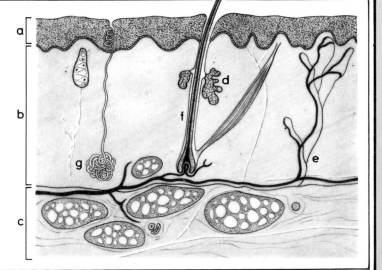

© DIAGRAM

If you go to a beauty salon or health farm, you will be able to choose from a wide range of treatments which you cannot duplicate at home because of the complex and expensive machinery required. As with all professional beauty treatments, you should make sure that the beauty therapist operating the equipment is properly trained.

VIBRATORY TREATMENTS

Gyratory vibrators have a similar effect to a good manual massage, but act much more quickly and effectively. The back, shoulders, arms, buttocks, and legs are the areas that are usually treated; the abdominal area is sometimes treated, but only with great caution. These vibrators should never be used on the face, kidney area, bust, or any parts of the body where there is little underlying fat, as they can cause damage.

The therapist has a choice of several different types of vibrator applicator or "head," each of which has a different effect. The first head to be used is usually made of sponge – a round sponge for the back and shoulders, and a specially shaped sponge for the arms and legs. The sponge heads are intended to relax you and so prepare you for treatment with the other applicators. A ball-headed applicator may be used gently over your abdomen, or a "pin-cushion" applicator (made of rubber with short rounded rubber spikes) on areas of rough or pimply skin. Applicators with heavier prongs are used on areas where there are large muscles or deposits of fat, such as the thighs, buttocks, and the sides of the waist.

Gyratory vibrator treatments
1, 2 A shaped sponge applicator is used on the legs. The therapist always moves the applicator up the leg, toward the heart.

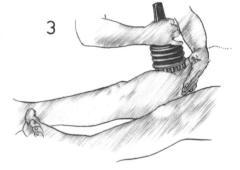

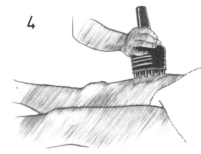

3, 4 A heavy prong applicator is used to massage the solid tissues of the thighs. The applicator is moved in circles over the thighs, again always working upward toward the heart.

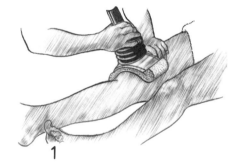

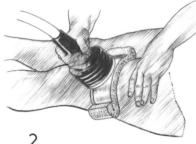

5, 6 A ball-headed applicator is moved in gentle circles over the abdomen, and with firmer pressure on the sides of the waist.

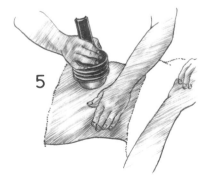

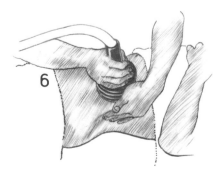

HIGH FREQUENCY TREATMENTS

An indirect high frequency treatment combines an electrical treatment with hand massage. You will be asked to hold a piece of the apparatus called a saturator electrode. The beauty therapist will place one hand firmly in contact with your body (usually on your thigh) and will use the other hand to turn on the electricity and to adjust the controls that govern the strength of the current. Once the current is strong enough for you to feel a pleasant tingling sensation, the therapist will use both hands to massage you. At the end of the treatment the therapist will turn down the current using one hand only, before switching off the machinery and removing the other hand from your body. It is very important that the therapist keeps at least one hand in contact with your body at all times during the treatment, or the flow of the electric current will be broken. The treatment should leave you feeling very relaxed, with a sensation of deep warmth in your body tissues.

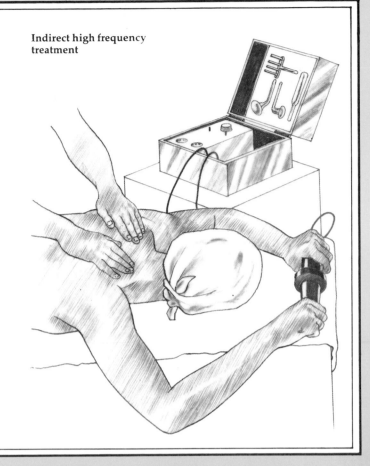

Indirect high frequency treatment

IONTOPHORESIS

This treatment makes use of a galvanic current – an electric current that flows in one direction only, from negative to positive. (The ordinary alternating current in the mains supply changes direction at regular intervals.) Beauty therapists use the galvanic current to introduce water soluble cosmetic preparations right into the upper layers of the skin, instead of just onto the surface. The current flows through electrodes which are covered in lint pads soaked in the treatment solution. Rubber elasticated straps are used to hold the pads firmly against your body, and the therapist then turns up the current until you can feel a prickling sensation. The treatment will last for a maximum of 20 minutes.

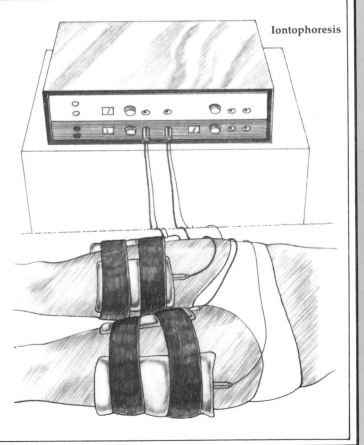

Iontophoresis

81

VACUUM MASSAGE

In this treatment, clear plastic suction cups are placed on your body. When the electric current is switched on, the cups act like small suction pumps, pulling up the flesh underneath them and then releasing it. Because the cups are transparent, the therapist can see exactly what is happening and adjust the suction power accordingly. The cups are available in various sizes, depending on the area to be treated. Large cups are used on areas where there are fatty deposits (such as the thighs and buttocks) and smaller cups on the less well-covered areas (such as the back and shoulders). The exact treatment will depend on the design of the vacuum massage equipment being used. With some types several suction cups can be used at the same time: the cups are left in place on your body during treatment, and each cup sucks and releases in turn. With other designs the therapist massages you with a single cup, moving it over the area to be treated with rapid, stroking movements. Vacuum massage can be used on any part of your body where there are layers of fat. If it is used on areas where there is little or no fat, it can overstretch the skin. It should never be used near your kidneys, as the strong suction may damage them, or on bruised areas or areas where the veins are broken or varicosed. Bruising can be caused if too high a level of suction is used, or if a treatment session is allowed to go on for too long.

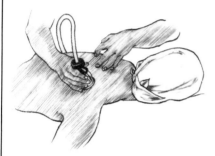

Vacuum massage on the back

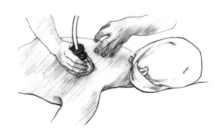

Vacuum massage on the shoulders

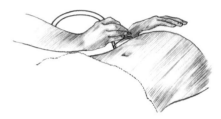

Massaging the sides of the waist

MUSCLE CONTRACTION TREATMENTS

These treatments use a faradic current to simulate the effects of exercise and tone up your muscles. A faradic current is one that is produced in regular surges: as it flows through the electrode pads that are strapped to your body, it stimulates your muscles to contract and relax. When the current is first switched on, you will feel a slight tingling in your muscles. The strength of the current will then be increased until you can feel a definite, rhythmic, muscle movement. Each of the muscle groups treated will contract and relax over 1000 times in an average treatment session, which lasts about 35 minutes.

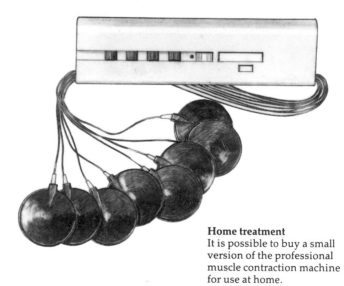

Home treatment
It is possible to buy a small version of the professional muscle contraction machine for use at home.

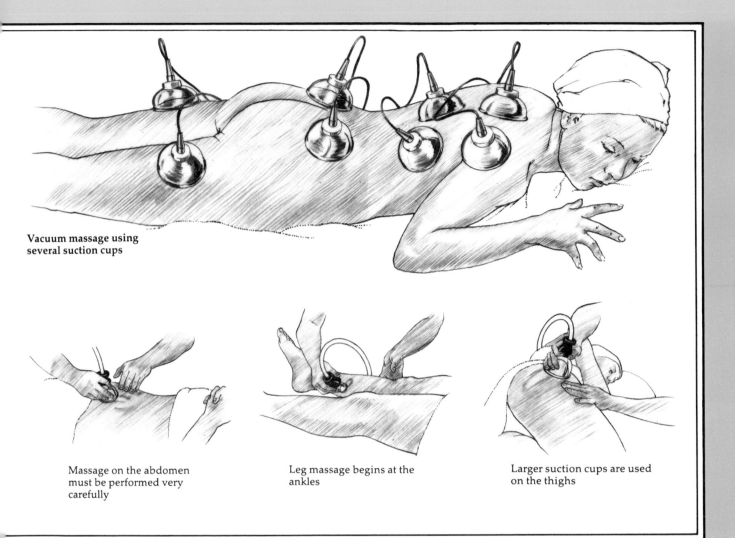

Vacuum massage using several suction cups

Massage on the abdomen must be performed very carefully

Leg massage begins at the ankles

Larger suction cups are used on the thighs

Muscle contraction treatment

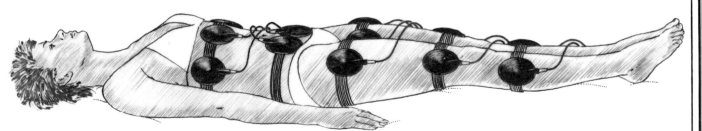

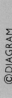

Breast care

Apart from being an obvious and outward sign of a woman's femininity, breasts have an important part to play in her sexual and reproductive life. Each breast consists of a number of lobes, rather like the segments of an orange. These contain tiny ducts through which milk is conveyed to the nipple during breast feeding. The lobes are surrounded by fibrous tissue and encased in fat. Breasts contain no muscle which means that exercise alone cannot alter their shape.

SIZE AND SHAPE

The size of your breasts depends on your overall body size, your body's natural hormonal levels, and to some extent on genetic factors. The breasts develop at puberty in response to hormone stimulation and many women notice an increase in their normal breast size before a period, during pregnancy, and while taking the contraceptive pill. Most women have one breast larger than the other. The size of the breasts has nothing to do with the ability to breast feed.

Some women with small breasts choose not to wear a bra regularly but for most women the choice of bra can make a significant difference. Choose a bra which is well fitting but not restricting, with enough room for your nipples. Small busts can be augmented by padded bras; underwiring can help support heavy or sagging breasts. All pregnant women are advised to wear a bra to give extra support to their enlarged breasts.

EXAMINING YOUR BREASTS

The breasts should be examined every month, preferably just after a period. The first part of the check involves simply looking at the breasts to observe any changes that may have taken place; the second involves feeling, or palpating, your breasts to check for the presence of any lumps.

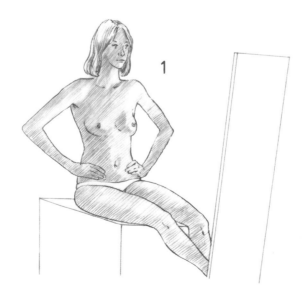

1 Sitting naked before a mirror, you should look for any change in the shape, size, or colour of the breast or nipple, any puckering or dimpling of the skin, and any discharge from the nipple.

2 Lie down, your left shoulder supported on a folded towel, and place your left hand behind your head, keeping your elbow flat. With the right hand, gently feel the left breast, starting at the outer edge.

3 Continue to examine the breast in the same way, working in a clockwise spiral toward the nipple.

4 Examine the area around the nipple and gently squeeze the nipple itself to check for any discharge.

5 With both arms now by your side, feel the armpit to check for lumps. Repeat on the other breast and report anything unusual to your doctor immediately.

COSMETIC SURGERY

Breast augmentation is one of the most popular cosmetic surgery operations. The breast is enlarged by inserting a soft silicon gel implant or an inflatable implant filled with saline solution. The operation involves a general anaesthetic and a two day stay in hospital. The incision is made around the areola, where it heals leaving an almost imperceptible scar. The implant itself is placed deep in the breast against the chest wall. The stitches and dressings are removed after about 10 days and there is usually little discomfort. Results are good and cases of infection or rejection are rare. The breasts look and feel natural and breast feeding is still possible.

Breast reduction is a more complicated procedure and involves a longer stay in hospital. There may be bruising and discomfort after the operation and scarring is more extensive. There may be a loss of sensitivity in the nipple and the ability to breast feed may be impaired. The incision is made around the areola and is continued down to where the breast meets the chest wall. Skin, fat, and tissue are removed and the nipples are resited. Breast uplift involves similar techniques to breast reduction except that only skin is removed. This has the effect of improving the contours of the breasts, but it cannot fill out breasts that have shrunk due to age, fluctuations in body weight, or pregnancy.

IMPROVING THE BREASTS

The simplest thing you can do to improve your bust line is to check your posture. A rounded back and hollow chest will give you an unflattering profile; simply standing up straight with your shoulders held back, but still relaxed, can make an immediate difference to your overall appearance. Unfortunately, some women feel very anxious about the size and shape of their breasts and bad posture represents their attempt to conceal what they regard as a problem.

Exercise alone cannot change the shape of the breasts but it can strengthen the supporting muscles and certainly encourages better posture. Losing or gaining weight affects the breasts just as it does the rest of the body so small changes in breast size can be achieved by diet. Major changes in breast shape and size require cosmetic surgery.

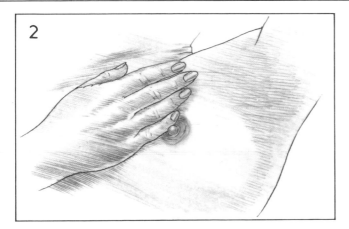

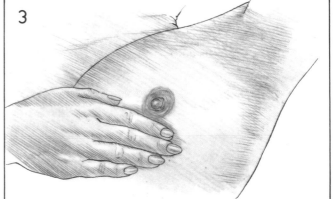

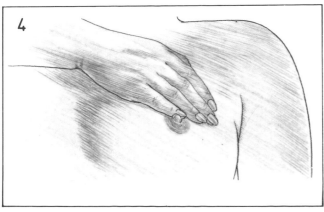

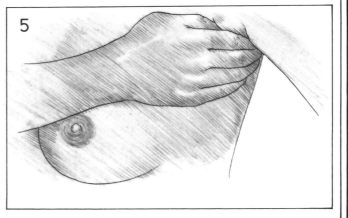

Hand care

Your hands are in action almost all day long and are relied upon to perform many different tasks. They are an important medium of self-expression and can be the focal point during a conversation so it is necessary to take good care of them, to keep them healthy and attractive, and to avoid unsightly problems. Few of us have the elegant hands we would like but it is possible for every woman to make the most of the hands she has by giving them a little regular care and attention.

WASHING
Always remove jewellery before washing your hands. Discoloured areas can be treated by rubbing a cut lemon over the skin. All-over grease and grime is better removed with a heavy duty cleanser. Careful drying is important as hands left wet can become chapped and are open to infection.
Always apply a hand cream after washing.

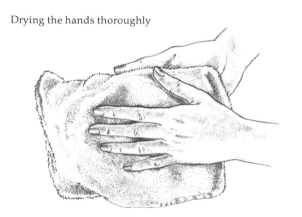
Drying the hands thoroughly

PROBLEMS
Many problems affecting the hands can be prevented. Some of the most common causes and treatments are given here.
Circulatory problems
The hands, like the feet, are particularly susceptible to problems arising from poor circulation. By the time the blood reaches the hands, the flow of blood through the arteries can become quite sluggish. Blood flow is slowed even more by cold and the hands may take on a purplish colour and may be affected by chilblains – painful, inflamed swellings on the fingers. It is essential to keep the hands as warm as possible and to keep the blood flowing as efficiently as possible; hand massage or exercises (see pp. 88–89) can be a great help.
Tingling fingers
It is common for pregnant women to experience a tingling sensation in their fingers. The condition may also result from nervous overbreathing. Very rarely, tingling fingers can indicate a blood disorder or disease of the nervous system, so if the symptoms persist, or if you are taking the contraceptive pill, it is important to consult your doctor.

Trembling hands
This problem is commonest among elderly people and is often a natural part of the aging process. Sometimes the onset of arthritis aggravates the problem by impairing manual dexterity. Trembling can also occur during illness, especially if there is a fever, and at times of stress and nervousness.
Sweaty palms
Fear or excitement can trigger the sweat-producing mechanism. Washing the hands regularly and dusting with talc can help control the problem.
Dermatitis
Hands are particularly vulnerable to this allergic skin reaction because of their exposure to irritants such as washing or cleaning products. The rash may take the form of dry, scaly skin patches or small blister-like lumps. Avoiding causes of allergy is the only real treatment for this problem.

HAND CARE

If hands remain in water for long periods, or if they are subjected to immersion in very hot or very cold water, much of the natural oil in the skin is sapped away and dehydration results. For this reason, rubber gloves should be worn whenever possible. Since the rubber makes the hands sweat, it is important to choose gloves with a cotton lining, or to wear rubber gloves for short periods only.

Some women find that a barrier cream containing water-resistant silicone helps protect their hands if applied before some household jobs.

For "dry" jobs, cotton gloves may be worn. They allow the skin to breathe naturally and if you apply a little moisturising cream before putting on the gloves, your hands can have a beauty treatment while you work!

Always wear special gloves for gardening; they keep the hands and nails clean and protect them from cuts and scratches.

It is important to establish the habit of applying hand cream morning and night, and after washing. A jar of hand cream by each sink and washbasin is a useful reminder. If your hands are exceptionally dry, you may like to apply a richer moisturising cream at night when it has several hours in which to restore softness to your skin.

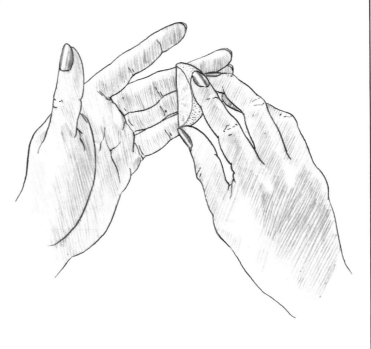

Using a lemon to remove stains

Warts

These small hard growths are fairly common on the hands. They are possibly caused by a virus. Warts often vanish without treatment but if they are large and unsightly you may wish to use a wart-removing solution or to have them removed by your doctor.

Rough hands

Severely roughened hands can be treated by immersing them for a half hour in warm olive oil. Alternatively a moisturising face mask may be used.

Calluses

These are areas of skin hardened by friction. You can smooth them away by rubbing gently with a pumice. Afterwards rub in lots of hand cream. Repeat this treatment daily until the callus has disappeared.

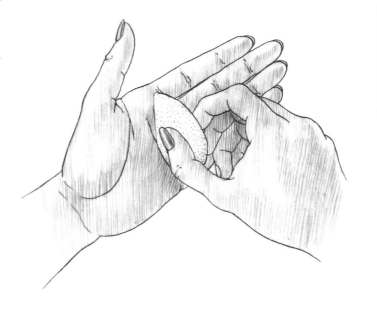

Using a pumice to remove a callus

©DIAGRAM

Hand massage and exercises

HAND MASSAGE

Every time you apply hand cream you are massaging your hands. The vigorous action stimulates the blood flow to the skin and this is as important as the softening qualities of the cream itself. From time to time you can treat your hands to a full-scale massage.

1 Warm your hands by shaking them gently. If they are very cold, try immersing them in warm water.

2 Apply cream to the palms of the hands. For a night-time massage choose a rich moisturising cream; for daytime a barrier cream containing water-resistant silicone may be more suitable. Rub the cream well into both palms.

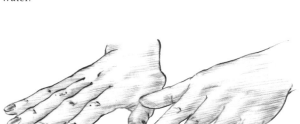

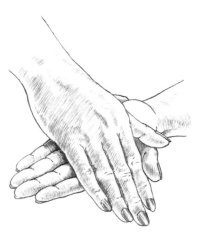

HAND EXERCISES

By practising these exercises every day you can help make your hands more supple and expressive, increase their strength, and improve the circulation.

1 Clench both fists tightly, hold for a second (**a**), then open out your fingers as wide as possible (**b**). Repeat six times.

2 Put your hands palm down in front of you with the fingers straight and pressed tightly together (**a**). Then spread your fingers, as in the previous exercise (**b**). Repeat six times.

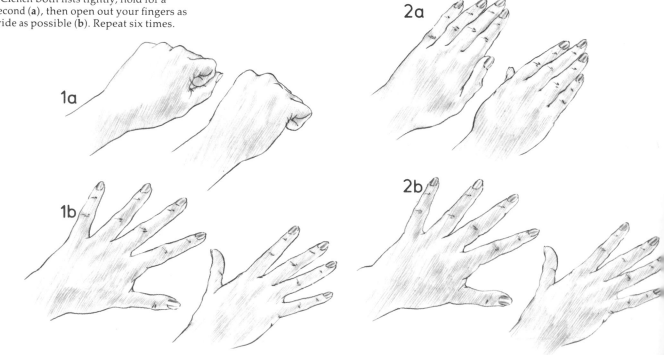

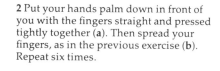

3 Now rub the cream into the backs of the hands. This is generally the driest part as the skin is most exposed.

4 Imagine that you are putting on a pair of gloves and work down each finger slowly. Concentrate on the joints and the sides of the fingers.

5 Massage the whole of the hands with smooth downward movements from the fingers to the wrists. Relax your hands and feel the tension easing from them.

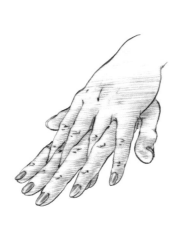
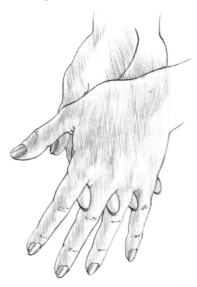
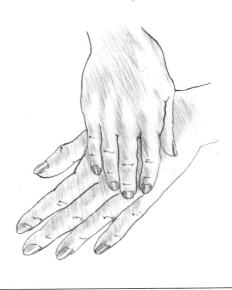

3 Allow your hands to dangle loosely from the wrists (**a**). Keeping the hands and wrists relaxed and limp, lift up the arms from the wrists (**b**). Drop the arms and repeat the movement six times.

4 Stretch out your arms in front of you and rotate your wrists 10 times outwards (**a**). Then rotate them 10 times inwards (**b**).

5 Spread your fingers and, using your thumbs, make a wide circling movement (**a**). Repeat using your forefinger (**b**), and then with each finger in turn.

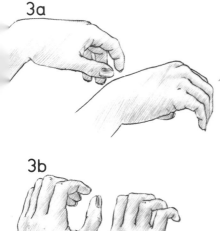
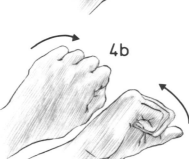
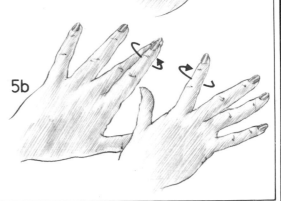

Nail care

Whether you wear your nails short or long, varnished or plain, it is important to keep them looking their best at all times. Protect them with gloves from excessive exposure to cold, wind, water, detergents and other chemicals; concentrate on the cuticles whenever you apply hand cream; and include a regular weekly manicure in your beauty routine. A nail grows at the rate of about 2mm each month and can take more than six months to grow from root to tip. For this reason, any damage to the nail bed or matrix will be obvious for several months in the growing nail. Similarly, treatment to improve the condition of the nails will show results only gradually.

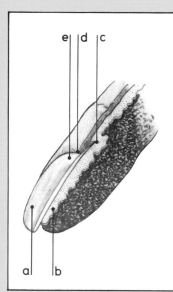

Structure of the nail
The nail plate (**a**), the visible part of the nail is, in fact, dead. It consists of layers of keratin, a hard, enamel-like substance, and lies above the nail bed (**b**). The most important part of the nail is the matrix (**c**) at the base of the nail plate. From here the nail cells grow and push forward. Sometimes the top of the matrix is visible as the half moon or lunula (**d**). The nail bed is protected by a thin strip of skin around the nail plate, known as the cuticle (**e**).

NAIL PROBLEMS
Included here are the causes of, and treatments for, some common nail problems.

Ridges
Ridges on the nails are usually the result of damage to the matrix or nail bed caused by rough treatment of the cuticles. More rarely, they can occur after a blow to the nail. If the cuticles are left alone the ridges should grow out.

White spots
These are normally the result of a bang or knock to the nail bed. They too grow out in time.

Cloudy or stained nails
Leaving polish on your nails for long periods, or the prolonged use of an alcohol-based polish remover are the most common causes of this problem. Let the nails go free of polish for a while, and massage them with a special preparation containing lanolin and protein.

Splitting and brittle nails
A problem for many women, brittle nails are usually caused by dryness. Wear rubber gloves when you can to protect your nails from water and detergents, and apply a hardener to the nails to discourage splitting.

Cracks
These appear if you file the nails too low down at the sides. A commercial nail repair kit (see p. 96) can be used while the cracks grow out.

Hangnails
These unsightly slivers of hard skin or nail are caused by cutting or pulling at the cuticle or biting off bits of skin surrounding the nail. They can be quite painful. Hangnails should be trimmed carefully with cuticle clippers or scissors. Avoid them altogether by releasing the cuticle from the nail; push the skin back gently as you dry your hands. Apply cuticle cream regularly to keep your cuticles supple.

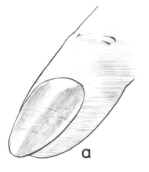
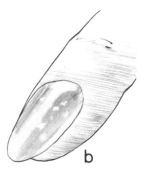
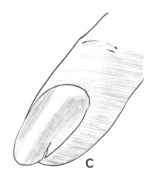
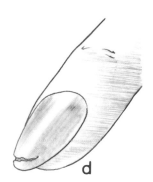

a   b   c   d

NAIL CARE HINTS

Look after your nails in the following ways.
● Clean your nails gently every day to prevent the build up of dirt.
● Manicure regularly (see pp. 92–93).
● Avoid using any metal nail care instruments as they can scratch the nail's surface or damage the nail bed or matrix.
● Wear gloves for heavy or dirty work, or if the hands are to be immersed in water for long periods.
● Treat your cuticles with care. Do not pick at them or push them back roughly or you may damage the entire nail area.

NAIL BITING

This is a nervous habit that often dates from childhood. In severe cases, the shape of the nail is so badly damaged that normal growth is never resumed. Painting the nails with a bitter-tasting substance may discourage nail biting, though some people find that simply taking extra care of their hands and nails can help them break the habit.

Sore skin

Picking at uneven cuticles or the rough edge of a nail can make the skin around the nail sore. Keep the nails well trimmed and the cuticles soft and smooth.

Whitlow

A painful, boil-like infection growing under or near the fingernail is known as a whitlow. If it appears on the nail bed it may disturb nail growth. Bathing and poulticing can be soothing but if there is an accumulation of pus the whitlow may need to be lanced under a local anaesthetic.

Common nail problems
a Ridge
b White spot
c Split
d Crack
e Hangnail
f Whitlow

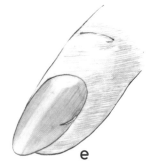

NAIL CARE EQUIPMENT

A considerable variety of equipment is available for looking after and grooming the nails.
● Emery boards can be bought in varying sizes and degrees of coarseness. A small, fine board is probably the most useful for general use. Boards need to be replaced regularly.
● Wooden sticks are useful for cleaning beneath the nail tip. Covered with a wisp of cotton, they can be used for applying cuticle creams and polish remover.
● A chamois leather buffer will give your nails an attractive sheen.
● Scissors and nail clippers should be used only when absolutely necessary. Cutting or clipping the nails can weaken them; shaping with an emery board is usually preferable. Careless clipping of the cuticles can cause hangnails and nail bed infection.
● Cuticle cream and cuticle remover help keep the cuticles soft and the nail bed healthy.
● Hand cream or lotion should be applied each time the hands have been in water.
● Nail hardener can be applied to strengthen nails that are inclined to split.
● Nail polish and polish remover are additional beauty aids.

Some useful aids
1 Emery boards
2 Cotton-tipped stick
3 Chamois leather buffer
4 Cuticle clippers

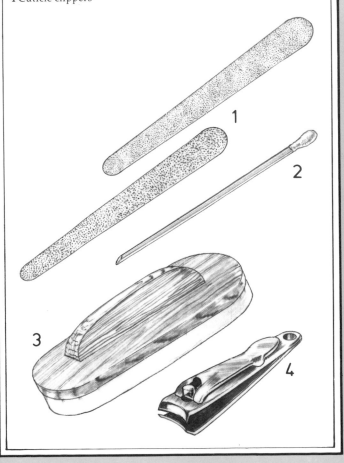

Manicure

Setting aside a half hour each week for a home manicure is an excellent way of keeping your nails in top condition. Between the weekly manicure sessions, nails should need little attention except perhaps cleaning with a soft brush and a wooden stick. Always avoid using a metal file for this job; metal can make scratches in the nail's surface, which then collect dirt. Remember to rub in lots of hand cream around the nails every time your hands have been in water.

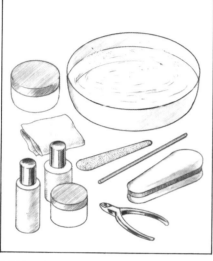

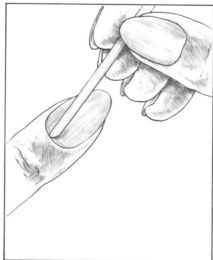

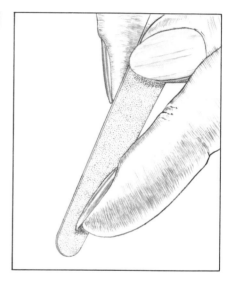

MANICURE ROUTINE

1 Begin by assembling all you will need: cotton wool, emery board, wooden stick, bowl of warm water, cuticle cream and remover, clippers, buffer, hand cream, nail hardener, polish remover, and polish.

2 Soak a piece of cotton wool in oily polish remover and hold it against each nail for about 20 seconds to dissolve all the polish. Sweep the cotton wool from cuticle to tip, never in the opposite direction.

3 With a fine emery board shape your nails to a smooth oval, filing from side to side and never to and fro. To avoid splits, do not file too low down at the corners of the nails.

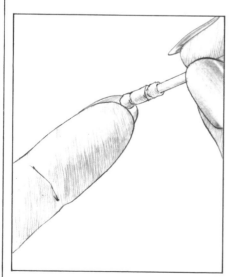

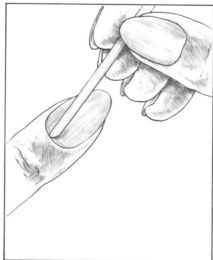

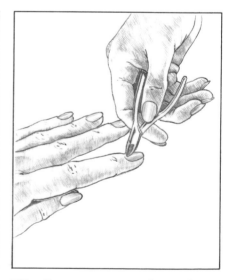

7 Wrap cotton wool around the pointed end of a wooden stick and gently clean out the nail tip. Be careful not to poke the stick into the skin beneath the nail.

8 Rub in cuticle remover, or apply special lotion from its applicator. Gently work around the cuticle to remove dead skin.

9 Use clippers to remove any hangnails or **dead skin** on the cuticle. This should be done only when absolutely necessary, as it is easy to cut the cuticle itself.

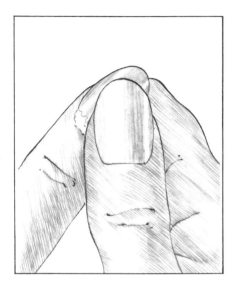

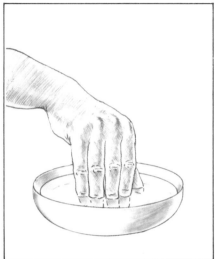

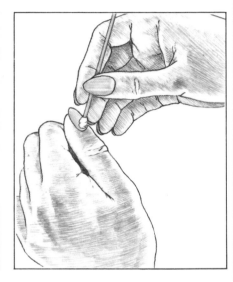

4 Rub a generous amount of cuticle cream into the nail and cuticle, using circular movements of the thumb.

5 Immerse the hands in a bowl of warm water for 3 minutes to soften the cuticle. Dry the hands on a soft towel and apply a little hand cream.

6 Ease back the cuticles with your fingertips. Dip a cotton-tipped stick into cuticle cream and use it to push back the cuticle all around the nail.

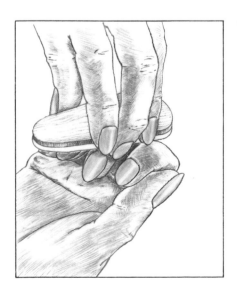

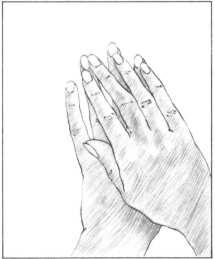

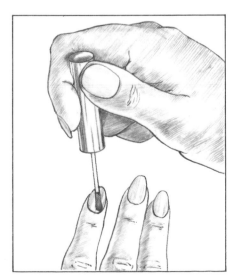

10 Encourage a healthy shine by buffing the nails with a soft chamois leather buffer.

11 Massage hand cream well into the hands from the fingertips to the wrist. Remove excess cream from the nails with a pad of dampened cotton wool.

12 Apply a nail strengthener if necessary, and allow it to dry. You are now ready to apply nail polish (see pp. 94–95).

Nail polish

Nail polish is a beautiful addition to well-cared for hands. It does, however, draw attention to your hands and nails, so if you plan to use polish regularly see that your nails are kept neatly manicured and your hands soft and smooth.

All nail polish and remover has a drying effect on the nails and if used constantly can rob the nails of valuable natural oils. For this reason it is advisable to leave the nails free of polish from time to time. Before applying any colour to the nails a basecoat should be used. This reduces any staining from the pigment in the polish. Two or even three coats of coloured polish should be used to give an even covering. The polish may be plain gloss or matt, or frosted.

A spray-dry aerosol speeds up the drying process and a hardener or sealer may be used to prevent chipping.

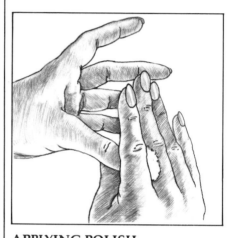

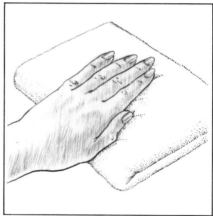

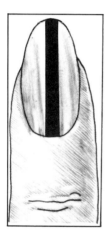

APPLYING POLISH

1 Remove old polish, using a pad of cotton wool soaked in oily polish remover. Wash your hands and check that your nails are neat, or give them a manicure (see pp. 92–93).

2 Rest your hand on a folded towel to keep it steady while you paint your nails. Begin by applying a basecoat.

3 Use four swift strokes. Make the first stroke up the centre of the nail, from base to tip.

4 Make the second stroke follow an arc around the nail bed.

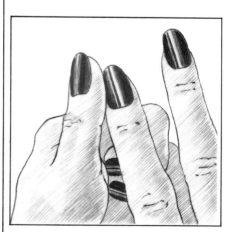

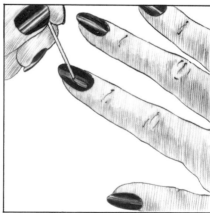

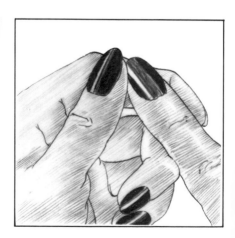

9 Free the nail edges.

10 Once the first coat of colour is dry, apply a second colour coat, making sure that any brush marks are evened out.

11 Free the nail edges.

USEFUL HINTS

Here are some hints you may like to consider when choosing and applying nail polish.

The most flattering shades to choose are the medium tones of coral and pink. Pale creamy colours and deep, harsh purplish-reds are more difficult to wear. Slightly coloured gloss, made by adding a drop or two of coloured polish to a bottle of clear, looks very attractive with a suntan.

To make your nails look longer and slimmer, leave a polish-free gap at the side edges of each nail.

You may like the effect obtained by leaving your half moons free of polish.

Remember that you can dress up your nails for a party by sprinkling a little glitter onto the top coat of polish as it dries, or by gluing a sparkling sequin onto dry polish.

Try to apply polish last thing at night so that it has several hours in which to harden.

Touch up chipped areas of polish rather than starting all over again.

Never apply polish near a heater or fire as it can cause the polish to "bubble".

Old, thickened polish can be thinned down by adding a few drops of remover.

To prevent the polish bottle cap from sticking to the bottle, smear it with a little petroleum jelly.

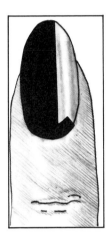
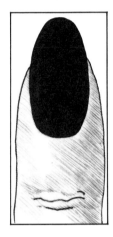
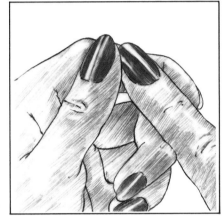
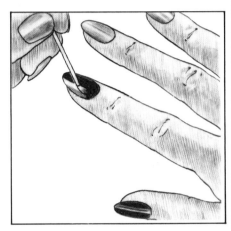

5 Cover one side of the nail with your third stroke, brushing from base to tip.
6 Cover the remainder of the nail with your fourth stroke, again from base to tip.

7 Work lightly around the tip of each nail with the thumb of your other hand to take away the build up of polish on the nail edge. This "freeing" of the nail helps prevent chipping.

8 Once the basecoat is dry apply the first coat of colour, as described in steps 3–6.

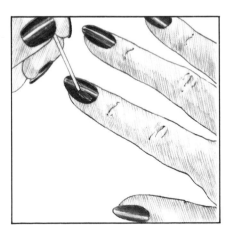
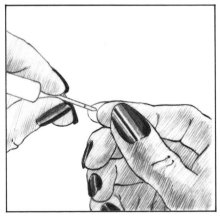
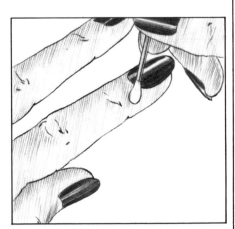

12 Once the final colour coat is dry, apply a clear top coat; free the edges.

13 If you want to, apply a hardener or sealer, brushing along and under the nail tip to seal the polish.

14 Remove any trace of polish from the skin, using a cotton-tipped stick dipped in remover.

© DIAGRAM

95

False nails

False nails can be invaluable for concealing split or broken nails, or for disguising ill-cared for nails. There are two main types of false nail – stick-on and brush-on. Stick-on nails come in sets of ten, can be applied at home, and can be reused many times. Brush-on nails consist of quick-hardening acrylic and are best applied professionally.

If you do not want to use a false nail for covering a broken fingernail, you may be able to patch it with a nail repair kit.

BRUSH-ON ACRYLIC NAILS

These are a very realistic form of false nail but can be difficult to apply. The surface of the nail is roughened to give a good key for the acrylic. Crescent-shaped moulds are placed under the edge of the nail tip. The acrylic solution is then brushed over the nail and mould and left to harden. The mould is then removed, and the nail is shaped and painted in the usual way. The false nail adheres firmly to the natural nail and grows out with it. Brush-on nails cannot be removed. There are sometimes growing out problems when the join between the false and the natural nail becomes visible. The nail must then be remoulded or filled.

NAIL-PATCHING KITS

These are useful for repairing broken nails. Repairs are available at salons but it is possible to buy kits for home use. These consist of special tissues and a quick-drying adhesive. Concealing a break can be a painstaking task and you should allow at least 15 minutes.

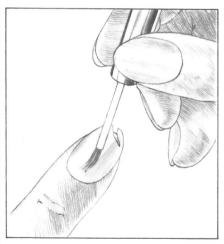

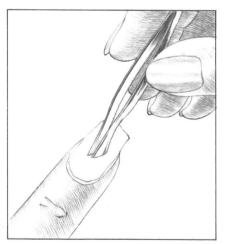

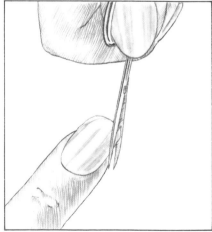

Nail patching procedure
1 First apply a basecoat to the whole fingernail, brushing it also onto the underside of the tip. Tear a tissue from the pack. Holding it on one forefinger, brush generously with adhesive.

2 Using tweezers or a wooden stick lay the tissue over the break in the nail and press it gently in place.

3 Apply adhesive to the underside of the nail tip. Fold the tissue over and press against the underside of the nail tip. Trim away surplus tissue. For extra strength, a second layer of tissue can be applied over the first. Apply nail polish as usual.

STICK-ON NAILS

Made of flame-retardant cellulose acetate, stick-on nails are the easiest false nails to apply at home. They can look very natural as long as you choose the right size and shape for your hands. They can be used singly or as a set.

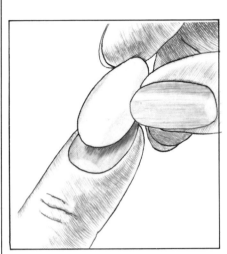

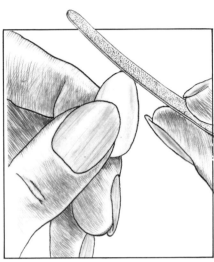

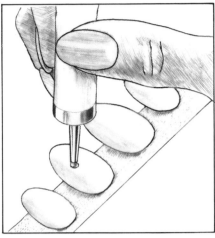

Using stick-on nails
1 Check that the nails are the right shape for you. If the curve is insufficient, soak the nails in hot water and then mould them carefully around a pencil or wooden stick.

2 Use an emery board to smooth away any rough edges on your own nails. File the false nails to the shape you want.

3 Apply a small amount of nail adhesive to the bottom half of the underside of each false nail. Leave them for 20 minutes.

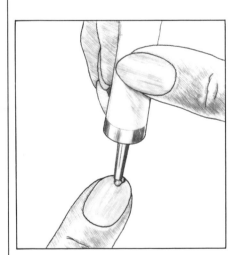

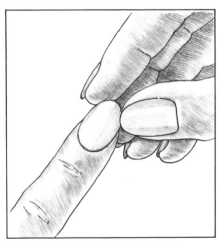

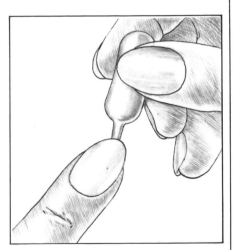

4 Gently release the cuticles from your fingernails. Apply a little adhesive to the centre of each fingernail from tip to cuticle.

5 Press the prepared false nail onto your fingernail, carefully slipping it under the loosened cuticle. Hold in place for a second or two and leave to dry for at least a half hour. Apply polish as usual.

6 To remove a false nail, apply a drop of adhesive solvent under the nail tip, using a cotton-tipped stick. Gently rock the false nail until it lifts off.

Foot care

It is not surprising that many people suffer from aches and pains in their feet. The feet are extremely complex structures, each with 26 bones, 19 muscles, and more than 100 ligaments; they take the weight of the whole body; they are responsible for the balance, movement, and manoeuverability of the body; and, being farthest from the heart, tend to have a sluggish blood supply. In addition to these factors, feet are usually hidden away in shoes and therefore easy to neglect.

Problems with the feet can affect the skin, muscles or bones. Causes include poor hygiene or lack of general care. Fungi, bacteria, and viruses all cause foot problems.

Apart from the discomfort in the foot itself, painful feet can have far-reaching effects. They can cause leg and back pain, postural problems, and fatigue.

Caring for your feet is vital and there are many simple things you can do to keep them healthy.

Pay attention to hygiene; wash the feet every day.

Change tights or stockings daily.

Choose well-fitting shoes for everyday wear; keep high heels for special occasions as they throw undue weight onto the bones of the toes.

Make sure that socks, tights, and stockings fit correctly; stretch them back into shape after laundering.

Take care with toenails; many avoidable problems result from careless cutting.

Give yourself a regular pedicure.

Treat any cut or other injury with antiseptic cream immediately.

See a chiropodist if you experience pain in one or both feet.

Remember that the state of your feet is always reflected throughout your whole body. If your feet hurt, it will be obvious to everyone. Prevent problems from arising by giving your feet the attention they deserve.

A DAILY ROUTINE

Taking care of your feet makes good sense whatever age you are. A minute or two of care every day and a regular pedicure will mean that you should discover any problem as it arises and be able to deal with it before it develops into anything more serious. A step by step guide to healthy foot maintenance is shown below.

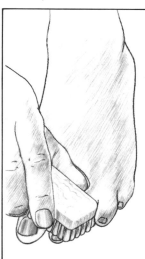

1 Immerse the feet in warm water. Wash each foot. Use a soft brush to scrub the nails.

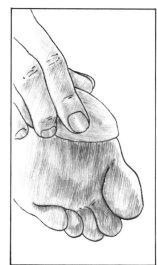

2 Rub any hard skin gently with a pumice stone.

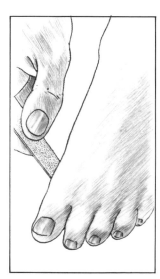

3 With an emery board remove any rough patches that might snag your tights or stockings.

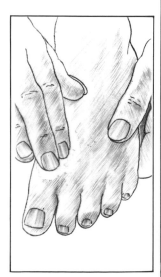

4 Dry the feet and apply a moisturising lotion, concentrating on areas of hard skin. Follow with a light dusting of talc.

TREATS FOR THE FEET

Tired feet can benefit from one or more of the following treats.

Make a whirlpool bath by sitting on the edge of the bath with your feet where the water enters the bath. Turn the water on at full pressure, first warm, then hot, then cold.

Give yourself a footbath by soaking your feet in hot water containing a handful of baking soda.

Rub swollen feet and ankles with an ice cube.

Lie with your feet higher than your head for a few minutes.

FOOT PROBLEMS

If you have a problem with your feet, deal with it immediately. Many things are simple to treat at first but can become more serious if neglected.

Ingrowing toenail

This painful condition occurs when the side of the nail grows down into the tender skin of the toe. It is caused by cutting the nails too low at the sides, rather than straight across. All ingrowing toenails need medical attention.

Athlete's foot

A highly contagious fungal infection, athlete's foot thrives on warm, damp areas of skin, especially between the toes. The skin becomes sore and itchy and forms scales that flake off. Creams or powders may be applied though sometimes treatment with an oral anti-fungal medicine is needed. Tights or stockings should be changed daily and the feet exposed to fresh air as often as possible.

Calluses

Calluses are areas of hard skin often caused by ill-fitting shoes. They can be removed by soaking the feet and then rubbing the hard skin with a pumice stone or special scraper.

Corns

Corns are small, round areas of hard skin with a cone-shaped central core. If the core presses against a nerve the pain may be severe. Small corns may be treated like calluses but large ones need professional attention. A ring-shaped plaster can ease pressure on a troublesome corn.

Chilblains

Poor circulation is thought to be the cause of these painful red lumps which can appear on the feet and hands in cold weather. Prevent them from forming by taking plenty of exercise to stimulate circulation. Avoid wearing tight boots or socks that might constrict the flow of blood to and from the feet.

Gout

The big toe joint is the most often affected by this painful condition, which is caused by an excess of uric acid in the blood. Overeating and drinking do not cause gout but can increase the uric acid level in the blood and so precipitate an attack. Medical advice is vital.

Verrucas

Caused by a virus, verrucas are painful, ingrowing warts on the feet. They may be cauterised or removed surgically.

Blisters

Friction can cause a fluid-filled blister to form. Small ones may be covered with a bandaid; large ones should be lanced with a fine sterilised needle to release the fluid. Keep the area clean to avoid infection.

Hammer toe

This is caused when toes are persistently bunched together in tight or pointed shoes. One or more toes eventually become permanently bent up at the joint and may need surgical correction.

Bunion

Bunions are painful, hard swellings at the base of the big toe. They originate from poorly-fitting shoes that push the big toe sideways and inward so that a bony lump is formed at the side. A pocket of fluid, or bursa, may develop between the bone and the skin. If you have a painful bunion, then seek medical advice promptly.

Fallen arches

Flat feet or fallen arches are not usually a problem but if the muscles that form the arch are weak and strained by carrying your weight, then your feet will ache. Arch strength may be improved by exercises and special sandals. You may find it comfortable to wear shoes with built-up arches.

Achilles tendonitis

It is possible to strain and inflame the Achilles tendon at the back of the ankle by wearing unsuitable shoes for long periods. Certain forms of exercise such as jogging can also exert undue strain on this and other tendons and muscles in the foot. Rest is the only treatment for this painful condition.

Foot massage and exercises

FOOT MASSAGE

Massaging the feet can be a delightful and relaxing experience. Massage helps to soothe sore and tired feet by improving the circulation. The massage is even more pleasurable if you use a herbal oil or body lotion. Concentrate on tender areas on the sole, heel, and side of the foot, especially if the feet have been rubbed by shoes that don't fit properly.

FOOT MASSAGE TECHNIQUES

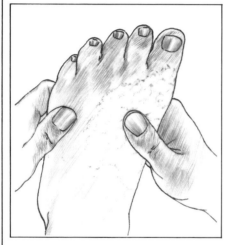

1 Massage the ball of the foot with both hands using firm, circular movements. Then massage the instep and then the heel.

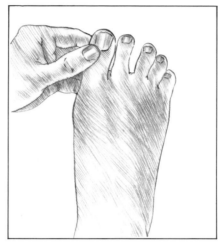

2 Press each toe firmly between the thumb and forefinger of one hand.

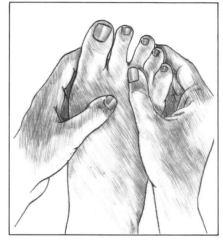

3 Again using thumb and forefinger, press firmly between the bones at the base of the toes.

SOME USEFUL EXERCISES

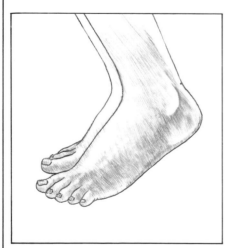

1 Stand barefoot with your feet together. Raise yourself slowly up onto your toes and down again. Repeat.

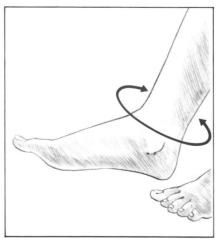

2 Sit on a chair with your legs crossed and one foot on the ground. Rotate the other foot from the ankle, first one way and then the other. Change your legs over and repeat the exercise.

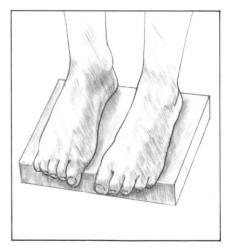

3 Stand barefoot on the edge of a big book. Curl your toes down over the edge, and grip as hard as you can. Relax and repeat.

EXERCISES FOR THE FEET

Feet spend much of their time squeezed into shoes so it is hardly surprising that they become sore and tired. Exercising them regularly will refresh them as it improves the circulation. One of the simplest and most effective forms of exercise is to walk barefoot. This natural exercise helps tone the whole foot. Exercise sandals can also be beneficial but some people find that wearing them for long periods can cause cramp in the feet and legs. An unusual and effective form of exercise for the feet is to put a layer of dried peas inside a pair of old shoes and then to walk in them for as long as you can bear!

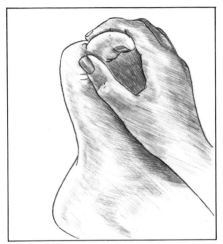

4 Clasp your toes with your hand, and bend them toward you. Then release them and repeat.

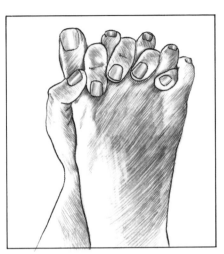

5 Slip your fingers between your toes, as illustrated. Bend your foot down, and then push it up.

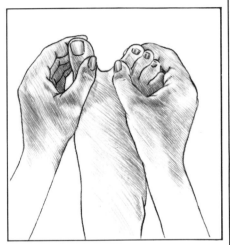

6 Use both hands to pull each toe gently away from the next one.

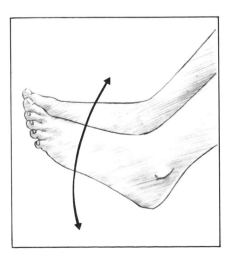

4 Sit on a chair with your legs stretched out in front of you and your feet raised from the floor. Move your feet up and down from the ankles.

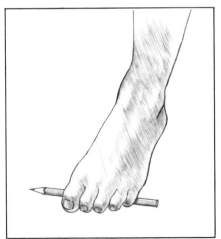

5 First clench your toes into a fist, and then try to spread them to make a fan. Relax. Then try to pick up a pencil with your toes.

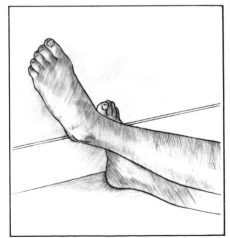

6 Lie on the floor with your feet against a wall. Use your toes to "walk" as far up the wall as you can. Stay in that position and relax for one minute. Walk down again. Relax and repeat.

©DIAGRAM

Pedicure

Your feet need and deserve a regular pedicure. They receive very rough treatment and will certainly benefit from any extra care you give them. Finding time once every two weeks to give them a full pedicure will increase your comfort and will certainly improve the appearance of your feet.

A professional pedicure is a real treat but with a little practice it is possible to achieve good results on your own feet at home.

You will find that a pedicure is particularly valuable when summer sandals reveal feet that have spent the winter in warm tights and heavy shoes. Choose nail polish colours carefully; pale pinks that tone with the skin are more flattering than vivid reds or purples.

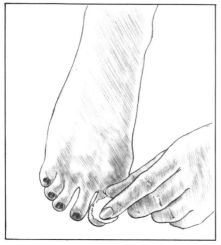

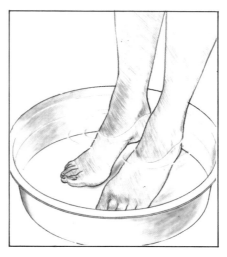

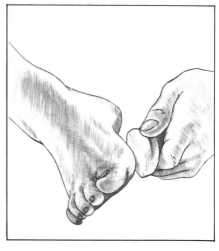

PEDICURE PROCEDURE

1 Use cotton wool soaked in remover to get rid of all traces of old polish. Sweep the cotton wool up the toenail from cuticle to tip.

2 Soak your feet in a bowl of warm water, or sit on the edge of the bath and let your feet soak in the tub. Wash each foot in turn with water and scrub the nails with a soft brush.

3 Use a pumice stone on any hard skin. For very rough patches try a paste or liquid skin remover. Obstinate areas of hard skin may need the attention of a chiropodist.

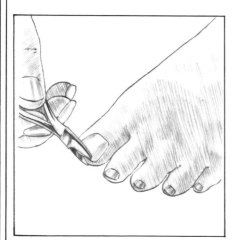

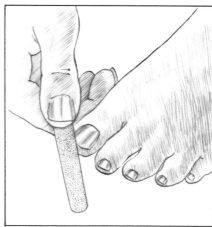

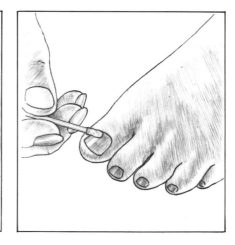

7 When necessary trim your toenails, cutting straight across. Nail clippers give a better shape than scissors.

8 Smooth any rough nail edges with an emery board.

9 Apply cuticle cream to the nail, working around the sides and base of the nail and gently easing back the cuticle with a stick to reveal the half moon.

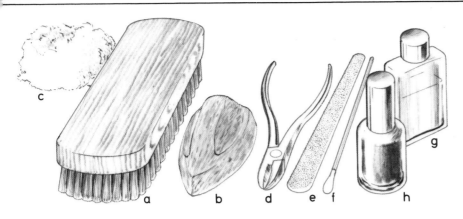

Pedicure equipment
Useful equipment for a
pedicure includes the
following.
a Soft scrubbing brush
b Pumice stone
c Cotton wool
d Nail clippers
e Emery board
f Cotton-tipped stick
g Polish remover
h Polish

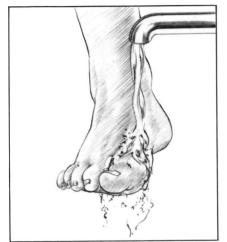

4 Rinse the feet with fresh, warm water.

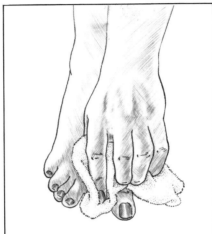

5 Dry the feet carefully on a soft towel, paying particular attention to the area between the toes.

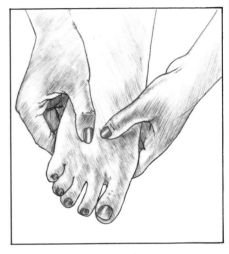

6 Massage in some moisturising lotion, concentrating on the areas where hard skin tends to build up. Massage up from the toes to the ankles.

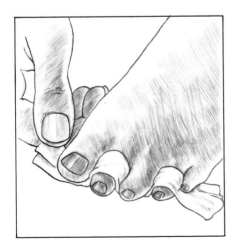

10 Separate the toes by twisting a tissue in and out between the toes. You can also use cotton wool or special pads to keep them apart.

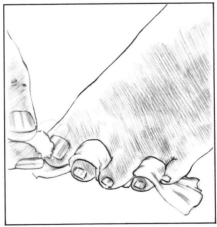

11 Apply a little nail polish remover to the toenails to take away any traces of grease remaining from the moisturising cream.

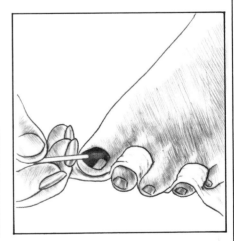

12 Apply a basecoat of polish using three broad strokes: one up the centre of the nail from base to tip, followed by two firm strokes to either side. Allow to dry, then apply a top coat of polish in the same way.

your face

Think of your face as the shop window of your self – your expression, the condition of your skin, and the sparkle in your eyes all tell people how happy and healthy you are. Fortunately today's skin care products mean that we can all quickly and easily give our faces the proper care that they deserve, however busy our lives. Cosmetic technology is extremely advanced today, offering products that are scientifically designed to suit today's modern woman and sorting out complexion problems with beneficial solutions.

Face shapes and skin types

Two of the most important factors in your appearance are the shape of your face and what type of skin you have. Your whole facial routine and approach to make-up will hinge on these factors – for instance you may need to compensate for an over-greasy skin, or want to play down a wide jaw. Beauty comes in all shapes and forms, and there are no hard and fast rules about the proportions necessary for an attractive face, but you will certainly find it useful to make a frank assessment of your good and bad points. Then you will be able to make the most of your assets and minimise your weaker features.

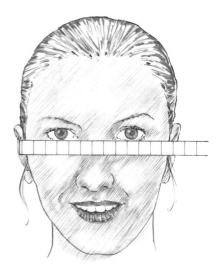

MEASURING YOUR FACE
Your face will be so familiar that you may not know if it is broad, long, or average. Tie or pin your hair back and then do some measuring.
1 Measure the length of your face from your hairline to the tip of your chin.

2 Now measure the widest part of your face, which will usually be across the top of your cheekbones. The classic oval face has a length equal to one and a half times its width; considerable variation from this implies that your face is extra long or extra broad.

FACE SHAPES
Checking the proportions of your face will help you identify your basic face shape.

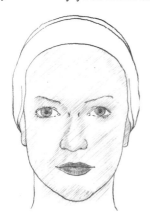

Heart-shaped face
This shape has a wide forehead and a long pointed jawline; use make-up to add extra width at the cheeks and jaw.

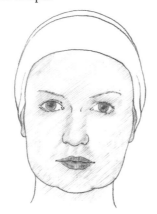

Square face
A square shape is characterised by a broad forehead and jawline. Soften the squareness with shading and a flowing hairstyle.

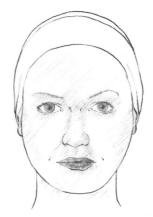

Round face
This shape is broad and short with rounded contours. Shade and highlight to bring out the bone structure and play down fullness.

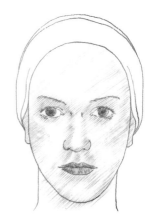

Long face
The frame of this face is narrow and long; style hair to add width, and use blusher on the cheekbones.

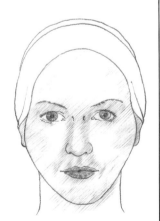

3 Check your profile by placing the rule against your nose and chin. If your mouth touches the rule, you have a receding or weak chin.

Oval face
This face is often classically beautiful, with no feature out of proportion.

Diamond face
This shape is wide at the cheeks with a narrow forehead and jaw. Use make-up to minimise width at the cheekbones.

SKIN TYPES

Skin type is determined by the level of activity of the sebaceous glands under the skin of the face. Whatever your skin colour, your skin will be one of four basic types. Take careful notice of your skin's characteristics, as you will need to choose your make-up and skin-care products accordingly. If you are not sure of your skin type, wash and cleanse your face and then leave it for a few hours without cosmetics; look for dry and oily patches after that time.

Oily skin
Oily or greasy skin has an overall shine. The skin is coarse and often sallow, with large open pores. Spots, blackheads, and acne are likely, as the sebaceous glands are over-productive, but oily skin stays looking young longer than any other types. Skin tends to be oiliest in a panel down the centre of the face.

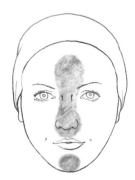

Dry skin
Dry skin looks dull and matt, feels taught, and is sometimes flaky. Because of its lack of sebum it is very vulnerable to extremes of temperature. Wrinkles may appear early, but spots and acne are not very common. Dry skin is usually most troublesome in the eye and lower cheek areas, here shown by shading.

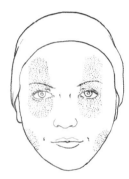

Combination skin
This is the most common skin type, with a central T-shaped panel of oily skin on the forehead, nose, and chin. The cheeks, throat, and skin around the eyes are dry. Black skins especially tend to have greater extremes of oiliness and dryness.

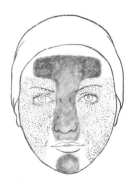

Balanced skin
This is the ideal we all aim for, but only a few achieve! The skin is fine in texture, smooth, and well-coloured. It rarely breaks out in spots, and looks youthful well into the thirties.

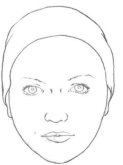

Skin changes

You may inherit a basic skin type, but its condition and needs change with your age and environment, and even with the different seasons of the year. Be ready to compensate for these extra influences, and adapt your skin care routine to keep your skin in top form.

TEENS

Puberty causes a great upheaval in the body's systems, and the hormonal changes taking place at this time affect the skin very noticeably. The sebaceous glands in the skin are stimulated to produce excess oil; this can cause problems if it blocks up the pores. Skin which was previously soft, perfect in texture, and even in tone may become coarser, develop enlarged pores, and erupt into blackheads or acne. These blemishes can be particularly distressing in the teenage years, but they can often be kept under control by careful skin care.

TWENTIES

This is the decade when your skin should be at its best, although it may begin to show signs of aging in the late twenties unless you take good care of it. Get into a good routine now and it will stand you in good stead for the rest of your life. Eat well and sensibly, making sure you include plenty of fresh fruit and vegetables in your diet. Also try to exercise regularly and get lots of fresh air, which will help your skin to "breathe". The first wrinkles often appear at around age 25, usually on the forehead and around the eyes. Skin that is dry and fragile will wrinkle earliest. Whatever your skin type, it is important always to keep your face well moisturised.

THIRTIES

Now is the time to guard against your skin drying out and aging prematurely. Activity of the sebaceous glands is slowing down, so it will no longer be necessary to concentrate so much on correcting oily skin. You will need to change your skin care routine as your skin matures: more emphasis is needed on gentle cleansing and moisturising, and less on toning and scrubbing. Deeper lines and bags under the eyes may appear, especially in women who have dry skin. The muscles around the sides of the face, along the jawline, and in the neck begin to lose tone, so keep your head high and work on facial exercises.

FORTIES

Some lines will now become permanently etched around your eyes, mouth, and nose. In the later forties your lips will begin to lose their fullness, a double chin may appear, and more wrinkles will show. Your skin will gradually lose its tone and strength, and the pores may enlarge. As the menopause approaches, the sebaceous glands produce less oil, so the skin becomes drier and more prone to flakiness. A form of acne, acne rosacea, may appear; its exact cause is not known, although alcohol, spicy foods, and stress seem to provoke it.

FIFTIES AND BEYOND

No matter how well you have looked after your face, it will now begin to show marked signs of aging. Collagen and elastin, the natural proteins that give the spring and firmness, begin to break down, so the natural lines on the face deepen, jaw and neckline sag, and the skin becomes drier. The menopause takes its toll as the production of estrogen decreases; the skin may develop itchy dry patches, and healing slows down. Little clusters of red lines forming small broken veins may appear on parts of the face. Deterioration in skin colour is often due to poor circulation, and can frequently be improved by massage and facial exercises.

ENVIRONMENT AND LIFESTYLE

Your surroundings and the way you live may contribute more than you realise to the condition of your skin. Moisturiser, enriching creams, cleansers, and toners are added to the outside of your skin to improve its condition, but what goes on inside your body will also affect your skin. Stress, poor diet, insufficient sleep, and lack of exercise will make your skin look dull, grey, and old. Outside agents can also affect your skin detrimentally. Pollution from exhaust fumes, factory smoke, and city living damage the skin's natural protective film, and can cause clogged and grimy pores. Extra cleansing is necessary in these cases. Lack of humidity in the air, for instance from drying winds or over-heated rooms, takes the moisture out of your skin; compensate with more moisturiser. Over-indulgence in sunbathing, alcohol, or smoking is also bad for the skin, and will cause it to age in advance of its due time.

Care Scrupulous cleanliness is vital to keep the skin free from excess oil and the pores unblocked. Treat the skin gently, however, as harsh scrubbing will damage it.

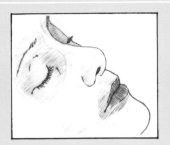

Using a face mask

Care Keep your skin clean and always make sure that any make-up is removed very thoroughly. Otherwise the pores will clog and the skin will look dull. Use moisturiser liberally, choosing a blend appropriate to your skin type; exfoliation creams and face masks will keep the skin clear of dead cells.

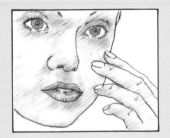

Applying moisturiser

Care Remove make-up gently with a cream cleanser. Moisturise with a rich cream and an eye cream at night; use a light moisturiser during the day, especially on your throat. Old skin cells tend to cling to the surface, so exfoliate regularly with exfoliating cream or a mildly abrasive brush.

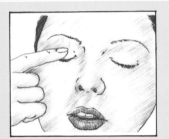

Applying eye cream

Care Remove make-up with a rich cleanser, and use only mild skin freshener rather than an astringent toner. Moisturise with a rich cream day and night and use eye and neck creams as well, as both these areas need extra pampering. Protect your skin well against the drying effects of the sun.

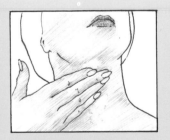

Applying neck cream

Care Use rich creams for make-up removal and moisturising, as well as eye creams, neck creams, and wrinkle creams. Use face masks and exfoliating creams very sparingly, and only the gentlest types for dry skin. Try not to expose your face to the sun; if you have to, use a high protection factor cream.

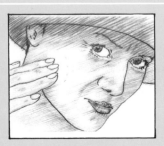

Protecting from the sun

Facial skin problems

The delicate skin of your face is exposed to everything that living in today's world can offer – extremes of heat and cold, dust, dirt, pollution, exhaust fumes, bacteria, and viruses. So it's not surprising that problems should sometimes occur! Some skin conditions, such as cold sores or chapped lips, only occur on the face. Others, such as acne or sunburn, may also occur elsewhere on the body, but present a particular problem on the face because that's the area that we have on show and so want to keep in peak condition. Here we look at some of the most common facial skin problems.

Freckles
These are usually very attractive, but some people find extensive freckling embarrassing. Freckles can be disguised by carefully applied make-up (see p. 126).

Brown patches
Brown patches on the skin are generally a result of the aging process; they cause most self-consciousness on the face and on the hands. They can be covered by make-up (see p.126).

Moles and birthmarks
Both of these are pigmented areas that can vary from the size of a pinhead to blemishes that cover large areas of skin. Most moles and some birthmarks are slightly raised from the rest of the skin. Large marks can be camouflaged with cosmetics (see p.126). Malignant melanoma, a particularly virulent form of skin cancer, can arise from a mole or birthmark; if a mark on your skin becomes tender or inflamed, increases in size, or changes in colour, see a doctor immediately.

COMMON SPOTS
Whiteheads
These are tiny cysts that occur just under the skin, particularly around the eyes. They can be removed by piercing them and then easing out the contents.

Blackheads
These are small plugs of sebum that clog up the pores and turn black on exposure to the air. Oily skin is particularly prone to blackheads; using an astringent toning lotion will help to keep them to a minimum. They can be gently removed to free the pores (see p. 117).

Acne
This is a distressing infection that can range from a few pimples to a thick covering of pustules, cysts, and craters across the face, neck, back, and chest. Home treatments include keeping the skin as clean and oil-free as possible, and avoiding fatty foods such as chocolate and bacon. Professional treatments include antibiotics, sunlamps, and skin peeling techniques (see p. 117).

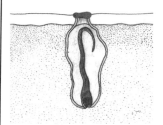

Blackhead
This cross section shows the blackened waxy plug blocking the skin pore.

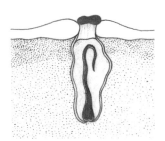

Acne
Here infection has set in after a pore has been blocked by a blackhead.

Sunburn

This is a common problem on the face because people like to have a healthily tanned complexion but forget that facial skin is delicate and needs special care. The nose and eyelids are often the first places to burn – the nose because it sticks out farther, and the eyelids because they are extra-delicate and because people often forget to apply protective cream there. Always use a suncream with an adequate protection factor, and moisturise your face thoroughly. If you do get sunburn, calamine lotion may ease the pain. (Also see pp. 76-77.)

Broken veins

These may occur with advancing age, or as a result of the skin being damaged by extreme weather conditions. The redness can be disguised with tinted cosmetics (see p. 126).

Wrinkles

Wrinkles are an unavoidable result of the aging process, occurring as muscle tone is lost and fatty tissue under the skin diminishes. Facial exercises (see pp. 118-119) and good skin care will keep them at bay for as long as possible; excessive smoking, drinking, and sunbathing will hasten their arrival. Face lifts (see p. 142) can eradicate the worst lines, but at considerable expense.

Bags under the eyes

These are usually caused by inadequate sleep. Although make-up can be used to disguise them, it is better to get to the source of the problem and have more sleep! As people get older, permanent bags form under the eyes as the skin loses tone and starts to sag.

Cracked and chapped lips

These are a result of the skin on the lips drying out. They can be relieved (and prevented) by applying a lip gloss.

Unwanted hair

This may occur on various parts of the body (see pp. 74-75), but can be particularly embarrassing on the face. The most usual sites are the upper lip and the chin. Because of the sensitivity of facial skin, waxing and shaving are not recommended; the only satisfactory way of removing unwanted facial hair is by electrolysis. This involves inserting a fine needle into the hair follicle and applying a low-powered electric current to kill the root of the hair. If facial hairs are very fine they can be bleached with a specially formulated preparation to make them less noticeable.

Cold sores

Caused by the herpes virus, cold sores occur as angry red patches around the mouth. The virus remains dormant in the body until triggered into activity by for example illness, injury, or sunlight. Cold sores disappear on their own and little can be done to speed up their rate of healing.

Boils

These are extremely painful bacterial infections. They are most common on oily skin, and may be a result of acne or may occur independently. The boil should be poulticed until it bursts and should then be cleaned carefully. Boils can be very disfiguring during their active phase, and can leave scars

Warts

These are rough, unpleasant-looking but painless skin growths believed to be caused by a virus. They can be particularly unsightly on the face, but can easily be removed surgically.

Sebaceous cysts

Developing when a sebaceous gland becomes blocked, these are firm, round, movable lumps under the skin. Large or disfiguring sebaceous cysts can be removed surgically; otherwise they may need no treatment and often disappear of their own accord. If a cyst becomes infected a doctor may give antibiotics and drain out its contents.

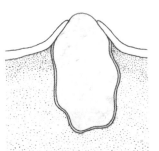

Boil
As shown here, pus builds up under the skin to give a boil its typical conical shape.

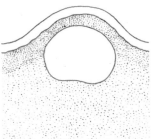

Sebaceous cyst
Here a lump is formed as the sac of a sebaceous gland fills with liquid or semi-solid matter.

©DIAGRAM

Basic skin care

Your skin care routine is really the key to good looks; make-up won't be a convincing beauty aid unless it is applied to a face that is in good condition. Your skin is a barometer of your health, and quickly loses its lustre and tone if you are at all unwell. Do what you can internally by getting plenty of rest, exercise, fresh air, and healthy food, then pay careful attention to the outside. The preliminaries here should never be skipped; each of them performs a different function that will contribute to the overall condition of your skin.

WASHING

The purpose of washing your face is to take off surface grime, excess sebum, and accumulated dirt, without upsetting the natural balance of your skin. Some people prefer cleansing their skin with water. Cleansers are available today that apply like liquid soap – but without the drying, harsh effects of soap – but *with* the benefit that they can be rinsed off with water. For a dry skin, it is better to use a gentle cream cleanser, that is lightly tissued off.

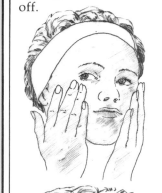

1

Washing procedures
1 Wet the skin with lukewarm, not hot, water and wash your face in light circular movements.

2 Rinse your face thoroughly with fresh lukewarm water.

3 Pat your face dry with a clean, soft towel.

2

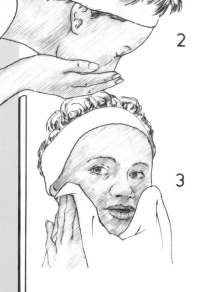

3

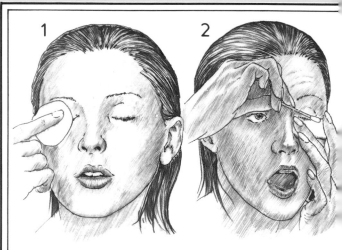

1   **2**

CLEANSING

Most cosmetic foundations, powders, and blushers are best removed with a specially designed cleansing cream or lotion, but usually the final particles need a deep clean with a cleanser. Many people with dry skin prefer to use a cleanser rather than washing their face. If you have an oily skin, choose a light, free-flowing cleanser; if your skin is dry use a richer, thicker one. Unless you are using theatrical make-up, avoid the very heavy cold creams.

TONING

Skin toners are pleasantly refreshing, and their evaporating and cooling action causes the pores to become temporarily smaller. Toners act as an additional cleanser on dirty or oily skin, and also remove any traces of grease left behind by the cleanser. The mildest forms are called freshners, or delicate toners. Astringents are the most powerful toning formulae, and are intended for oily skins. If you have a combination skin, don't apply strong toners to the dry areas.

BEAUTY PRODUCTS

If you have an oily skin, skincare products are specially designed for different skin types and should be chosen accordingly so that you compensate as much as possible for your skin's deficiencies. If you have a combination skin you will need to treat the oily and the dry parts differently if the end product is to be skin that looks balanced in tone and even in texture. For instance you may need a light moisturiser for the oily section and a richer, oil-based one on the dry areas.

MOISTURISING

Moisture is the most important element in skin chemistry. A moisturising cream will help to offset the evaporating effects of the environment – sun, wind, central heating, air conditioning and pollution. If used daily, especially under make-up, moisturiser will protect the skin, helping to seal in the vital natural moisture of the skin and acting as the perfect base for make-up.

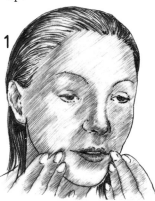

Applying moisturiser
1 With clean fingers, feel your skin gently for dry patches.

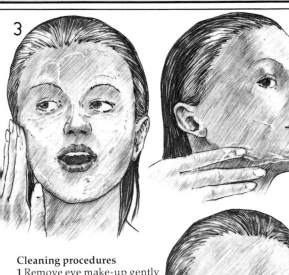

Cleaning procedures
1 Remove eye make-up gently with cotton wool pads soaked in special eye make-up remover.
2 Remove mascara by placing a moistened tissue under the lower lashes and stroking both sets of lashes together with cotton wool pads soaked in cleanser.
3 Apply the cleanser in circular movements, using your fingertips for cream cleanser or cotton wool for liquid cleanser. Start at the bridge of the nose and move out towards the areas around the eyes and cheeks.

4 Massage around the jaw and neck using upward strokes.
5 Remove the cleanser with cotton wool pads or paper tissues.

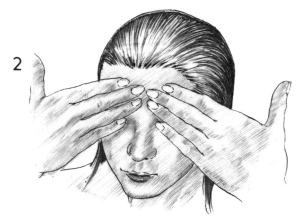

2 Smooth the moisturiser evenly over the required area with your fingertips, using upward and outward strokes and being careful not to drag the skin.

Applying toner
Immediately after cleansing, apply toner on a cotton wool pad – or pour a small amount of toner into the palm of your hand and splash it onto your face.

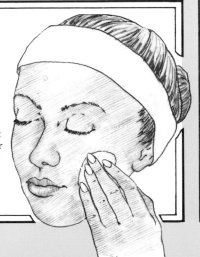

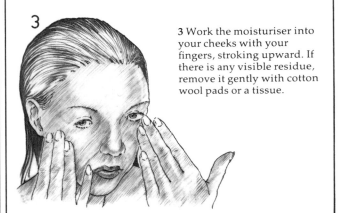

3 Work the moisturiser into your cheeks with your fingers, stroking upward. If there is any visible residue, remove it gently with cotton wool pads or a tissue.

©DIAGRAM

Special treatments 1

Your daily skin care routine is the most important factor in keeping your skin healthy and clean, but there are also special occasional treatments. These extras should be used occasionally to maintain your skin in tip-top condition.

The special treatments you need and the frequency with which you should apply them depend on your skin type, your age, and whether or not you have any problems such as acne or enlarged pores.

Treatments for oily skin

Since oily skin has a tendency to break out in spots, it needs efficient deep cleaning. You may need to use cleanser and astringent several times a day to keep the skin grease-free. Oily skin tends to suffer from enlarged pores, which in turn make it more liable to trap dirt and grease; the use of a cleansing face mask twice a week will help clear and tone the skin and draw out excess sebum from under the skin's surface.

Treatments for dry skin.

Dry skin should be gently cleansed morning and night, and kept supple with plenty of rich moisturiser. Skin foods, or nutrients, can be very good for maintaining a good skin balance; they lubricate the top layers of skin cells and keep them moist. Special eye creams and throat creams work on this principle and are important for dry and aging skin; use them liberally at night. Once a week use an exfoliating treatment to reduce flakiness; also, an occasional stimulating mask will encourage your skin to produce more natural lubricants.

Treatments for combination skin

To help even out your skin's texture, treat the skin on your nose, forehead, and chin as described for oily skin.

Treatments for balanced skin

You should have few problems with skin of this type; your main concern is simply to keep it clean and looking good with an occasional clarifying mask.

EXFOLIATION

Cleansing removes a certain number of dead skin cells from the face, but some tend to remain and clog the pores, giving the face a dull, grey look. Exfoliation is the process of sloughing off dead skin cells, which are then replaced by those underneath. If this procedure is done regularly, it will speed up the turnover and replacement of cells, which will help to open blocked pores and smooth the skin.

There are several methods of exfoliation to choose from.

● Brushes can be used with water. A shaving brush or a special complexion brush can be used to work over the entire face in a gentle circular motion.

● Facial scrubs can vary from almond shell to sunflower and birch leaves.

● Facial masks prepared with a special formula for exfoliation may also be used.

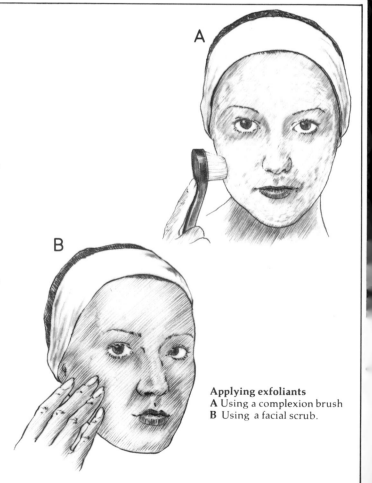

Applying exfoliants
A Using a complexion brush
B Using a facial scrub.

FACE MASKS

Face masks or face packs, in cream, gel, or liquid form, are applied to the skin and left to dry; they are then peeled or washed off. They stimulate the blood supply to the skin; this means that impurities, sweat, and excess sebum are drawn to the surface and removed with the mask. The extra blood flow also leaves the skin with a healthy glow, and makes it feel fresh and smooth. Face masks may reduce the effect of minor blemishes, such as enlarged pores or a slightly spotty skin, but they cannot deal with serious skin problems.

Types of face mask

● Clarifying masks are for oily skin. They are often based on clay, which is very absorbent and draws out excess oil. As the mask dries and tightens, the sebum and dead skin are combined with the mask and rinsed off at the end of the treatment.

● Stimulating masks are suitable for all types of skin. They act as a minor shock therapy, enlarging the surface blood vessels and bringing more oxygen to the skin, giving it a pink tone and healthy glow. They are usually in a brush-on, peel-off form.

● Moisturising masks are for dry to normal skins. These temporarily plump up the topmost layer of skin by causing the cells to enlarge slightly. This has the effect of smoothing out fine wrinkles, but only for a few hours. Moisturising masks are usually in cream form.

● Exfoliating masks are for all skin types, and are particularly useful for dry skins where the dead cells tend to cling to the skin's surface. A cream is applied and then left to dry on the skin; when it is rubbed off with the fingers, it takes the dirt and debris with it.

Applying a face mask
1 Tie your hair well back off your face. Using your fingertips or a brush, dot the face mask over your face, avoiding the hairline, lips, ears, and the area around your eyes.
2 Spread the mask evenly over the skin with your fingertips or the brush.
3 Remove after recommended time and follow with moisturiser or night cream.

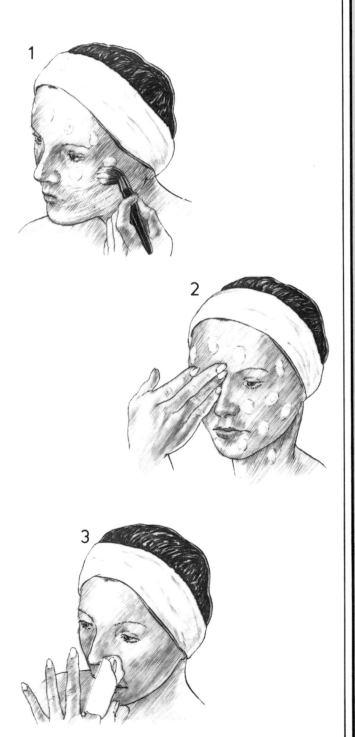

Special treatments 2

Every once in a while, you may feel that your skin needs an extra lift. Maybe you want to get it into its very best condition for a special occasion, or perhaps you just feel your face could do with some pampering in the middle of a busy lifestyle! Facials can be done at home, will take a little time, and work best when they combine beauty therapy with relaxation, so you should set aside a whole morning or afternoon. Because a facial of any sort opens the pores and cleans and clears the skin very thoroughly, your face will be very vulnerable to irritation or infection for a while afterward. After a professional facial treatment, give your skin a breather for a few hours; just apply a fine veil of moisturiser. Using make-up too soon will make your skin sore, and it will be difficult to remove it properly. However, after the waiting period you should find that your skin is in better condition than ever, and that your make-up has the best possible base in a clean and even-toned skin.

HOME FACIAL

Treat your skin to a home facial. The key is not to rush; the psychological effect of the relaxation is almost as important as the treatment itself. First do any little chores that might prey on your mind and stop your relaxing, then sit back and enjoy your beauty session!

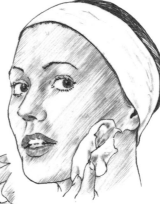

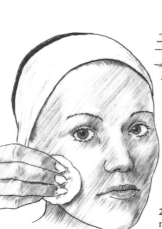

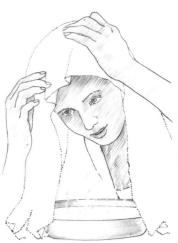

4 Have a facial sauna. Fill a bowl with boiling water and make a herbal infusion. Camomile is soothing, lavender purifying, comfrey healing, and rosemary stimulating. Put your head over the bowl, no nearer than 48 cm , and cover your head with a towel. Relax in the steam for five minutes at the most. If all this seems too complicated, soak a clean facecloth in hot water and hold it to your face for several minutes.

3 Apply a skin toner to remove any traces of cleanser or grease, and to tighten the pores.

2 Use a paper tissue to remove any cleanser that is left on your face.

Steps in a home facial
1 Cleanse the skin thoroughly with cotton wool and a gentle cleanser. Use strokes that go at right angles to any wrinkles – up and down strokes on the forehead, lateral movements around the lips, chin, and eyes.

PROFESSIONAL TREATMENTS

Beauty salons and in-the-home treatments provide a wide range of professional beauty care, from those designed to make your skin marvellous through to drastic treatments that will help remove acne scars.

● Facial massage helps to stimulate the blood flow to the skin and so improve its condition. You can do this yourself at home, but it is easier if a beauty therapist does it for you as it works best if you are fully relaxed. Moisturiser is massaged into the skin with firm movements.

● Deep cleansing uses a galvanic current to nourish and correct the balance of the skin. A special solution is applied to the skin, then rollers are moved lightly over the face to apply a current.

● Lymphatic massage uses small suction cups to stimulate the muscles under the skin.

● Heat lamps, ultraviolet or infrared, are used in many beauty salons. Heat lamps have, however, been implicated in the triggering of some skin cancers.

● Skin peeling is done by a plastic surgeon to remove badly scarred skin (usually caused by acne). Strong chemicals or a sanding mechanism remove the top layers of skin, and the face is raw and red until new skin cells grow. Do not expect the skin to be perfect in texture; it will also be very sensitive, and can develop pigmentation problems.

Deep cleansing

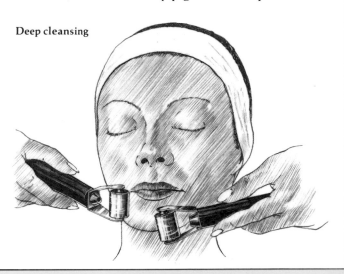

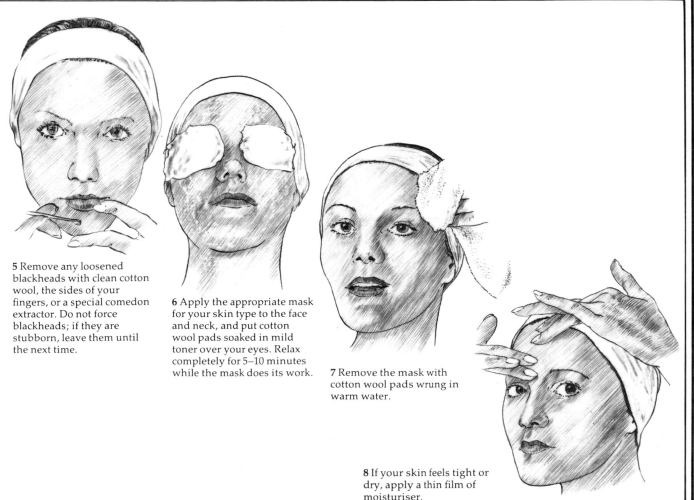

5 Remove any loosened blackheads with clean cotton wool, the sides of your fingers, or a special comedon extractor. Do not force blackheads; if they are stubborn, leave them until the next time.

6 Apply the appropriate mask for your skin type to the face and neck, and put cotton wool pads soaked in mild toner over your eyes. Relax completely for 5–10 minutes while the mask does its work.

7 Remove the mask with cotton wool pads wrung in warm water.

8 If your skin feels tight or dry, apply a thin film of moisturiser.

© DIAGRAM

Face exercises

It is well-known that regular exercise improves the muscle tone of your body and helps your figure to keep in good shape: exactly the same is true of your face. As you grow older, the layers of fatty tissue under the skin decrease and the muscles slowly lose their tone. The face starts to lose its firm shape and the skin begins to sag. In addition, stress, worry, or anger crease the face into unsightly wrinkles which can all too easily become permanent fixtures. Regular exercise will keep the muscles in your face firm and mobile, and will also help your face to relax physically and visibly after a stressful day.

FACE EXERCISES

Repeat this sequence of exercises several times each day.
1 Close your eyes and squeeze your face up tight. Relax.
2 Open your eyes wide and make a soundless "O" with your mouth. Relax.
3 Stick out your tongue and open your mouth in a silent scream. Relax.
4 Purse your lips, and move them to the left and to the right. Relax.
5 Open your eyes wide and grin from ear to ear. Relax.

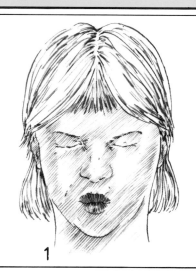

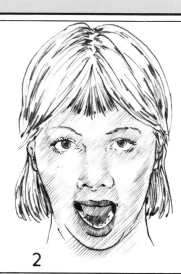

CHIN AND NECK EXERCISES

Repeat this sequence of exercises several times each day.
1 Begin each exercise by sitting up perfectly straight with good posture.
2 Bend your head forward, stretch your neck muscles. Return to your starting position.
3 Stretch your neck back with your mouth in a pout, your lower jaw thrust up and out. Straighten up.
4 Puff out your cheeks and circle with your head and neck, first clockwise and then counterclockwise.

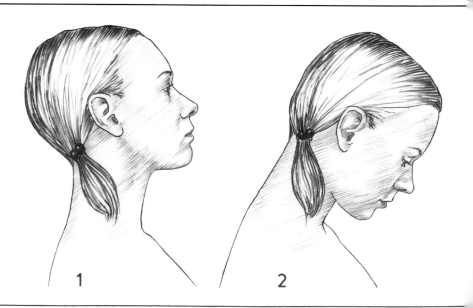

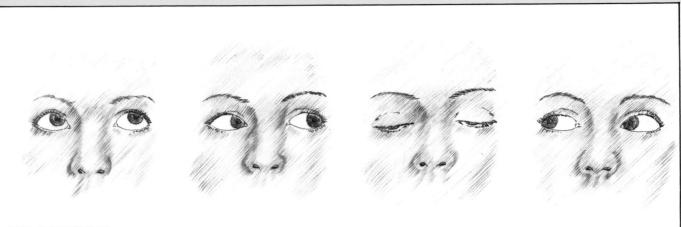

EYE EXERCISES
Relax your eyes by holding your head
completely still and rolling your eyes,
first clockwise and then counterclockwise.

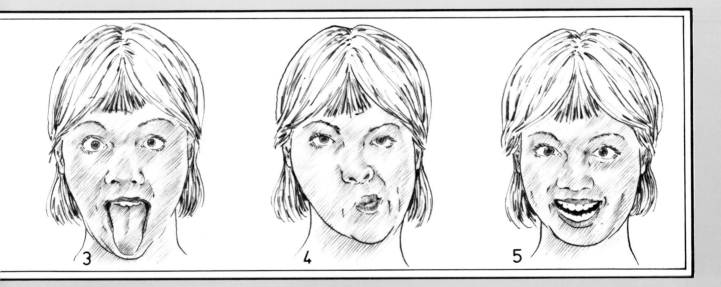

3

4

5

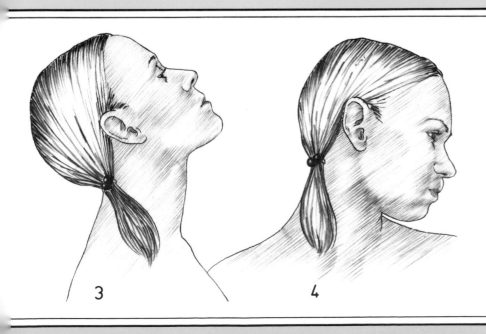

3

4

Cosmetics and equipment

Imagine your face as a canvas: cosmetics are the colours that will bring that canvas alive. You don't need a lot of expensive cosmetics in every colour of the rainbow; a few well-chosen ones for different occasions, and the right equipment to apply them, will serve you much better. Cosmetics should be chosen to match your natural skin tones, so that the look you create complements your features rather than appearing artificial. Within these guidelines you will want a selection of different types of cosmetic – bases (foundation and powder), contouring colours (shaders, highlighters, and blushers) and colours for your eyes and lips. Some colours will be chosen for daytime use or for wearing with particular clothes; for evenings you will probably want a selection of stronger, more vibrant colours that will show up well in artificial lighting.

Storing

Heat, light, and moisture can all damage cosmetics: lipsticks can melt, colours fade, and eyeliners and mascaras dry out. It's best to keep your cosmetics in a drawer or make-up case, arranged into sections so that you don't need to sort through all the eye shadows every time you want a lipstick. Remember to close all containers after use, and your cosmetics should stay in good condition.

BASIC EQUIPMENT

Some basic standbys will be invaluable for helping you achieve a professional, finished look to your make-up.

● Tissues will be needed for cleansing routines, for correcting mistakes, for blotting lipstick, and for keeping your hands and working surfaces clean.

● Cotton-tipped sticks are handy for removing smudges, blending shadows, and softening pencil lines. They also make good applicators for powder eye shadow.

● Dry cotton wool is perfect for applying toner and for dusting off excess face powder or powder eye shadow. Cotton balls are convenient, but a roll will work out cheaper.

● Sponges can be either natural or synthetic; it's good to have a stock of several for applying foundation. Clean and rinse them regularly.

● Powder puffs will be needed for loose and compressed face powder; soft swansdown puffs are particularly useful for loose powder.

● Eyebrow tweezers, scissors, eyelash curlers, and a cosmetic pencil sharpener will all come in handy too.

1 Cotton-tipped stick
2 Cotton ball
3 Sponge
4 Powder puff
5 Eyebrow tweezers
6 Scissors
7 Eyelash curlers
8 Cosmetic pencil sharpener

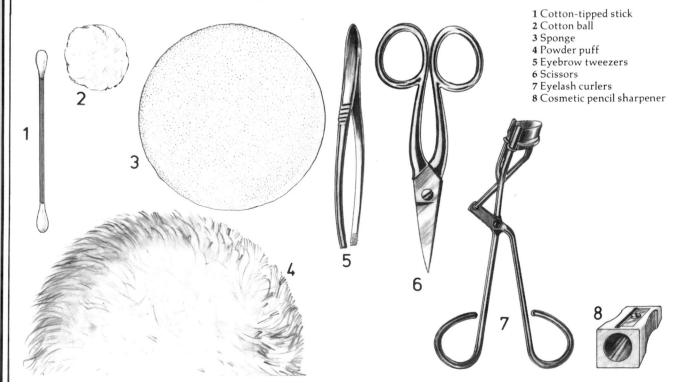

Allergies

Allergic reactions to make-up are rare: perhaps only 1% of users develop allergies to substances used in cosmetics. An allergy is a complex immunological response to a particular substance, and may be severe; the sufferer may experience rashes, blotches, sore patches, itching, or sneezing. Cosmetics described as hypoallergenic usually minimise these reactions. Many more people, however, are sensitive to a particular product without actually being allergic to it. Some cosmetics may make your skin feel sore, or tight, or itchy, or may leave it unpleasantly dry and scaly. This kind of reaction is more common among people who have fair skin, especially those who have fair or red hair. People with dry skin also tend to be more sensitive to some cosmetics, and sensitivity can increase with age as the skin becomes drier. If you often encounter sensitivity to make-up, use gentle, unperfumed, hypoallergenic cosmetics as far as possible. If any cosmetics provoke an allergic or sensitive reaction, read their labels carefully and see if you can detect any common ingredient that you should avoid in future.

Hygiene

Hygiene is important when using cosmetics: the skin of the face is sensitive and can easily be adversely affected by dirt or germs. Never borrow another person's cosmetics, or lend out your own. Make sure that your fingers and hands are very clean before you begin making up; a clean fingertip is often is often a better make-up applicator than a brush. Sponges and brushes can easily harbour bacteria, especially if they are left lying around; keep them clean by frequent washing in water and a mild detergent, and stand brushes upright in a pot to dry.

BRUSHES

Brushes for make-up come in all shapes and sizes. They are necessary for precision work around the lips and eyes, and also for applying light dustings of shader and powder eye shadows.

● Contour brushes are big, fat, soft brushes used for applying powder blushers, shaders, and highlighters.

● For eye make-up you will need several brushes, each for a separate range of colours. Choose from round or pointed brushes, or chisel-ended ones which make sharper lines.

● Sponge-tipped applicators are useful for loose eye-shadow powders, or for applying colour beneath the eye.

● Eyeliner brushes are small and fine with pointed tips; they are used for drawing fine lines or for applying small dots of colour.

● A lip brush is a chisel-ended brush, usually with a lid or a retractable head to stop it collecting dirt. Clean it by wiping off excess lipstick with a tissue and then rubbing in cleansing cream; wipe it clean with a tissue.

● An eyebrow brush is for training the brows into shape and for removing excess powder.

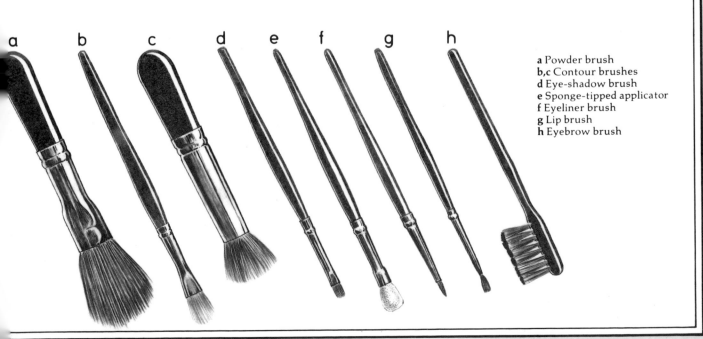

a Powder brush
b,c Contour brushes
d Eye-shadow brush
e Sponge-tipped applicator
f Eyeliner brush
g Lip brush
h Eyebrow brush

©DIAGRAM

Foundation and powder

Good make-up begins with an even, well-applied base, and this is produced by careful use of foundation and powder. The foundation provides the background tone and colour, and the powder used to set the foundation so that it doesn't streak or smear.

The colouring of your foundation and powder is very important, and should match your own natural skin tones. If your skin is very white, or pink and white, you can use pale foundations with a tan, honey, or pink tint. If your skin tones are more sallow, or suntanned, go for tan, beige, olive, or occasional peach shades – pink tints will look unnatural on your skin. If your skin is black or very dark, you can get away with dark tones of browns or reds.

FOUNDATION

Foundations come in several forms. Liquid foundation, in bottles, gives a light coverage and is suitable for fine or young skins in good condition. Most foundations are slightly thicker and come in tubes or pots – these are easier to apply, and give a more substantial coverage. Solid foundations, which come in cake form, are really only needed for badly blemished skin, for instance a face scarred by acne.

Your face should be very clean and grease-free before you apply foundation; if there are any traces of oiliness, apply an astringent lotion first. To avoid clogging the pores with foundation, apply a moisturiser first; allow 5–10 minutes for this to be fully absorbed before you apply your foundation. Put a blob of foundation in the palm of one hand, or on the back of the hand, and use clean fingers or a dampened sponge to apply the foundation in even strokes to one part of the face at a time.

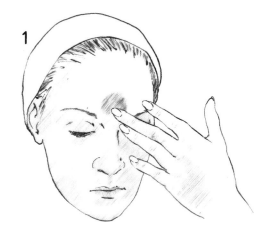 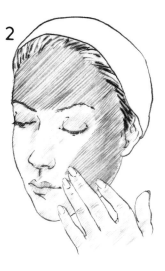 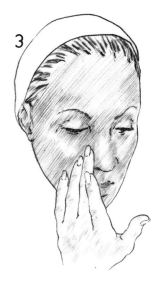

Applying foundation
1 Put a little foundation in the middle of your forehead and spread it with circular strokes to cover the entire area up to the hairline.

2 Work down from the temple, over the cheek, and under the eye; repeat on the other side of the face.

3 Put a dab of foundation at each side of the nose, and blend these over the nose and up over the eyelids. This will form a base for your eyeshadow.

Always test the colour of foundation or powder on your face rather than on your hand, as the tones are very different. If cosmetics are too light they will make your face look masklike; if they are too dark they will give it an unhealthy all-over flush. Remember that this is only a base to even out skin tones; colour and shading can be applied later.

5

4 Cover your chin, lips, and jawline, blending the foundation into the top of the neck to avoid leaving a sharp line.

5 Remove any surplus foundation from your neck, using the backs of your fingers in light upward strokes. Check closely in a mirror that the foundation is even. Blot all over with a tissue.

POWDER

Powder is essential to help set your foundation and to provide a grease-free surface for the rest of your make-up. It may be tempting to miss out on the powder, but it does give a more natural finish than bare foundation; the only time it can be left off is when you have used a bronzing gel as a base. Powder is available in two forms: loose and compressed. Loose powder gives a more translucent finish and is best for the first dusting after applying foundation; any surplus is easy to remove. Solid powder is more convenient and less messy to carry around, and is best used for quick repairs such as dusting a shiny nose. Because compressed powder tends to be thicker, it must be applied carefully and evenly to avoid a clogged or heavy finish.

The most popular powders are lightly tinted translucent ones. These provide a smooth matt finish, but allow the colour of the foundation to show through. If you use a non-translucent powder, choose a colour that is one shade lighter than your foundation.

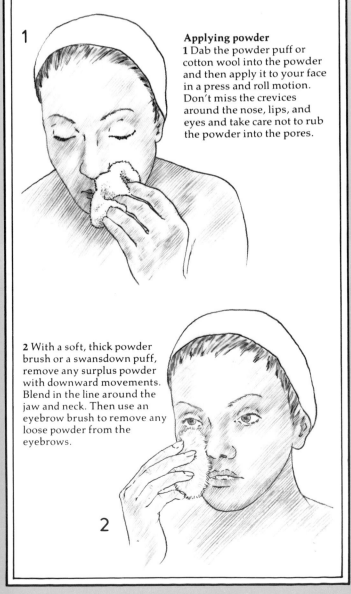

1

Applying powder
1 Dab the powder puff or cotton wool into the powder and then apply it to your face in a press and roll motion. Don't miss the crevices around the nose, lips, and eyes and take care not to rub the powder into the pores.

2 With a soft, thick powder brush or a swansdown puff, remove any surplus powder with downward movements. Blend in the line around the jaw and neck. Then use an eyebrow brush to remove any loose powder from the eyebrows.

2

© DIAGRAM

Highlighters, blushers, shaders

After you have laid a base colour with foundation and powder, you can emphasise the contours of your face with blushers, shaders, and highlighters. These bring life and shape to your face, emphasising bone structure and playing down faulty or irregular features. The basic principle is that colours paler than the skin bring features forward, while darker colours make them recede. Contour colour should always be subtle, blended with a light touch and not applied in harsh lines. Contour colours come as gels, creams, sticks, or powder. Gels and liquids give colour to the skin, with a light coverage that flatters tanned and even skin tone. Powder is the easiest to use, as layers of colour can be built up gradually. Look carefully at your face shape (see pp. 106–107) and decide which features you want to enhance and which you want to play down. Shader and highlighter work well together when chosen carefully. Blusher adds colour rather than shadow, and so can be of a richer hue, for instance a red blusher adding to shades and highlights in tones of tan or peach.

HIGHLIGHTERS

Use highlighters only on good features which you want to draw attention to, for instance well balanced cheekbones or an attractive bone structure around the eyes. The cheek and browbone form a natural frame for the eyes, and if these bones are highlighted they form a very dramatic setting for well blended eye make-up. Don't use a highlighter that is too pale; ivory, pale pink, or cream tones look better than white. Bronzes, golds, and deeper pinks look good on darker skin tones. Added shine or glitter intensifies the effect of highlighter, especially in strong sunlight or electric light.

APPLYING HIGHLIGHTER
A To emphasise the cheekbones, apply a line of highlighter from the outer corner of each eye, above the cheekbone, to the hairline.

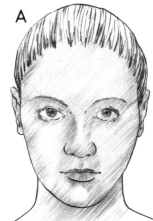

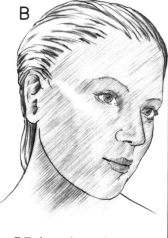

B To bring forward a receding chin, apply highlighter on the tip of the chin and blend it into the surrounding make-up.

BLUSHERS

Blushers are strong colours that add a healthy warmth and tone to the skin. Even faces that do not need contouring will look better with a little blusher, and mature skins are enhanced by soft shades of matt blusher. Oriental skins can be lifted with a dusting of a peachy tone, and black skins can be made really vibrant with reddish and plum shades.

It is important to place blusher properly. If the colour is too near the nose it can give the face a pinched look; always blend toward the hairline to give the face an open aspect. Blusher should be two tones darker than your skin tone.

Applying blusher
A To slim down your face, apply blusher just below the cheekbones and sweep it softly up and out toward the middle of your ear. To bring your chin forward, add a touch of blusher beneath the jaw.

B To give your face a healthy glow, use blusher over your cheeks, out toward your ears, and up beside your eyes and the outer part of your eyebrows.

C For a pretty, natural look, dab your blusher over the whole cheek and up to your temples.

D For evenings, use a stronger blusher and wear it high on the cheekbones to make your eyes look larger.

SHADERS

Shaders cause the part that they are applied to literally to recede into the shadows. Shaders can be used to emphasise good bone structure and to detract from pudginess or uneven features. Shading should be a subtle blending rather than obvious patches; use pinks, golds, peaches, and reds in daytime, and keep the darker browns for use under electric light.

Applying shader

A To emphasise cheekbones, use shader to draw a line under the cheekbone, from under the centre of the eye out toward the top of the ear. Draw a second line toward the bottom of the ear, then fill and blend.

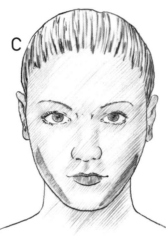

B If your nose is too broad, narrow the wide area with triangles of shader at the sides.

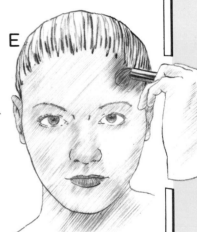

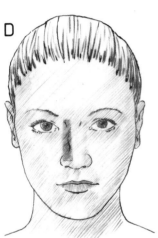

D If your nose is crooked, straighten its appearance by applying a little blended shader to the crooked side.

C Lift a heavy jaw by shading shapes just above the heavy part; blend well into the natural shades of the face and neck.

E To give a wide forehead a better proportion, apply shader to the temples and blend it in with the hairline.

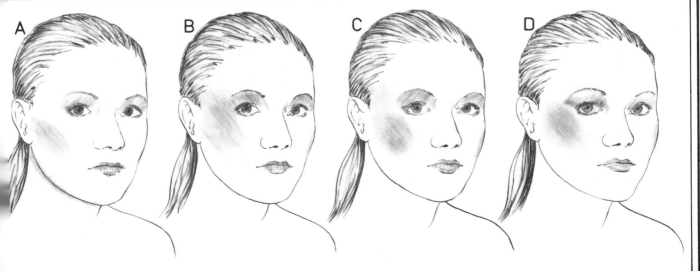

125

Camouflage make-up

Generally, make-up is used to enhance your good features, but it is also useful as a camouflage if you have blemishes on your face.

Blemishes can range from relatively minor conditions, such as broken veins or one or two spots, through to severe acne scarring or large birthmarks.

Because your face is on show all the time you are likely to be very conscious of any imperfections – probably far more conscious than anyone else.

Often the purpose of camouflage make-up is twofold: it plays down the imperfection, and it gives you more self-confidence.

The more severe the blemish, the more important it is to the wearer that the make-up is well set and will not streak, rub off, or wash off in rain. For very severe cases of scarring or very large birthmarks it is always worth seeking professional advice so that you can find the very best products for your condition. For less severe problems there are relatively simple camouflaging techniques that you will find simple to apply yourself after a little practice. Always make sure that the blemish cover is part of a full make-up and is well blended into the surrounding cosmetics. Do not moisturise before applying concealing make-up, which adheres best to a clean, dry skin.

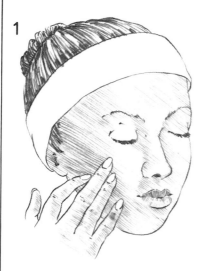
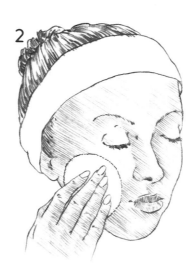

General cover-ups
This technique is useful for disguising large areas of slight discolouration, such as freckles, some pigmentation disorders, broken veins, age spots or a high colour.
1 Cover the entire blemish with a light coating of solid foundation, slightly paler than your natural skin colour. Blend the colour in well with your fingers or a slightly damp sponge especially around the edges.
2 Dust with powder to set. Now proceed with foundation and powder as usual, including over the camouflaged area.

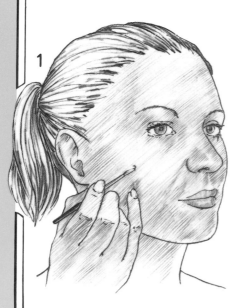
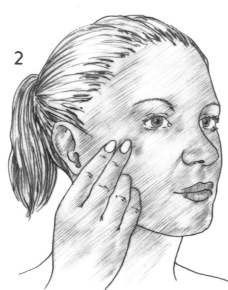

Covering spots
Almost every skin develops a few spots now and then, and it's useful to know how to play them down. Nothing is going to disguise a bad case of acne, but some people feel far more self confident if they use this spot-covering technique to make the worst blemishes less noticeable.
1 Using a wedge-ended brush, paint a little concealer onto the spot. The concealer should match your foundation exactly, otherwise it will only highlight the spot.
2 Continue with foundation over the rest of your face; don't touch the spot or you will expose it again. Then apply powder all over, including the spot.

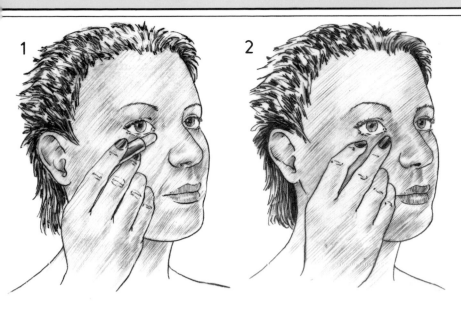

Concealing shadows

Concealer sticks can be very useful for playing down dark shadows under the eyes and between the nose and the mouth. Use a concealer that is a shade or two lighter than your foundation, otherwise it will deepen the shadow.

1 After you have applied your foundation, paint concealer over shadows you want to disguise. Use a brush or the tip of the concealer stick.
2 Blend in the edges with your fingertip or a brush, then apply powder as usual.

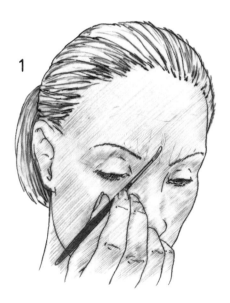
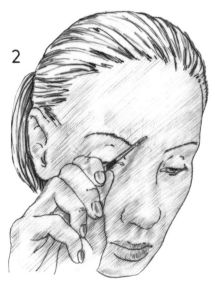

Covering acne scars

Many people's faces are marked by a few acne or chicken pox scars; the technique described here will make them less obvious. If your face is severely scarred by acne, the only method of significantly reducing the damage is skin peeling (see p. 117), but this is both too drastic and too expensive for many people; the technique shown here may help to play down the scars.

1 After you have applied foundation to your face, use a fine eyeliner brush to place a little light-toned concealer in each scar to lighten the shadow it casts.
2 Use ordinary powder on a small brush to set the concealer, carefully blending it into the foundation.

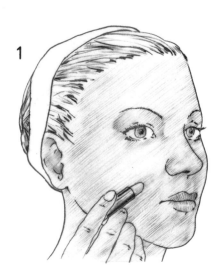
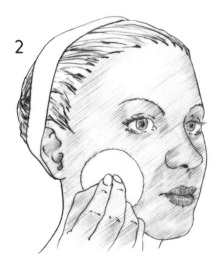

Covering birthmarks

Birthmarks can vary enormously in shape, size, colour, and texture, from small pigmented moles to portwine stains covering the whole face. This technique should help to minimise their effects.

1 Use a thick waterproof stick concealer with a high pigment content; liquid concealers will not be dense enough. Apply it to the entire discoloured area, and then smear and blend it around the edges with your fingertips.
2 Apply powder to set the concealer. Then continue with foundation and powder as usual. Raised marks tend to catch the light, so a gentle smudge of a slightly darker concealer may make the mark recede a little.

Lip make-up

Lip colour complements your other make-up and draws attention to a pretty mouth. It gives a boost to a complexion that may be a little dull, and so can be a particular asset to the older woman. Lipstick can be obtained in colours to suit the palest to the darkest skin, and to complement every kind of make-up effect from "nearly natural" to a dazzling evening look.

Although the solid stick is the most popular form of lipstick, good lip make-up can only really be achieved with a lip brush, as a stick is too wide to give a precise shape. Remember that the shape of your lips can be altered with make-up more easily than any other feature, so don't be afraid to experiment if you want a different look.

APPLYING LIPSTICK

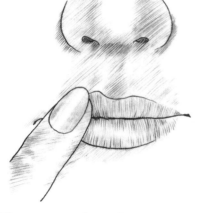 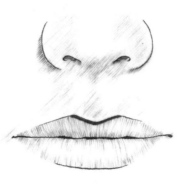 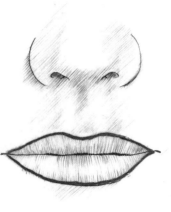

1 First prime your lips with a good base of foundation and powder.

2 Outline your lips with a lip pencil a tone or two darker than your lipstick shade. Define the bow on the upper lip with two precise strokes.

3 Continue the line on the upper lip, keeping your mouth closed and relaxed. Use short strokes, as they are easier than a continuous line. On the lower lip work from the centre out to the corners.

LIP SHAPES

A To give fullness to thin lips, apply foundation over the entire lip area and then outline with your lip pencil, just beyond the natural line of the lips. Fill in with lip colour in a bright shade, or use plenty of gloss.

B To play down full lips, apply foundation and then pencil your line just inside the natural lip line. Avoid glosses or bright colours, and blot off any extra sheen.

C Make droopy lips look more cheerful by covering the lip corners with concealer. Then use a lip pencil to extend the corners of the lip upward, and fill in with colour.

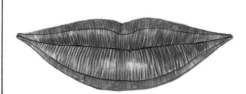 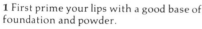 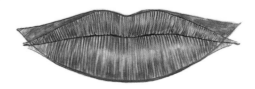

LIPSTICKS

As there are very few sebaceous glands on the mouth, the lips have a tendency to dry out, so lipsticks are generally softer than other cosmetics. Lip colourants are usually in stick form, but can also be bought as glosses or creams. Colours range from almost white to almost black, but most shades are dark or light tones of pink, red, beige, orange, peach, or plum.

Most lipsticks are based on a mixture of waxes, oils, and fatty alcohols, with pigments for colouring. If the pigment is allowed to reach the lips it will tend to dry them out; this is why a layer of foundation is so important. Because of the creamy consistency of lipsticks they tend to smear and smudge very easily; use a paper tissue to blot off excess lipstick after application.

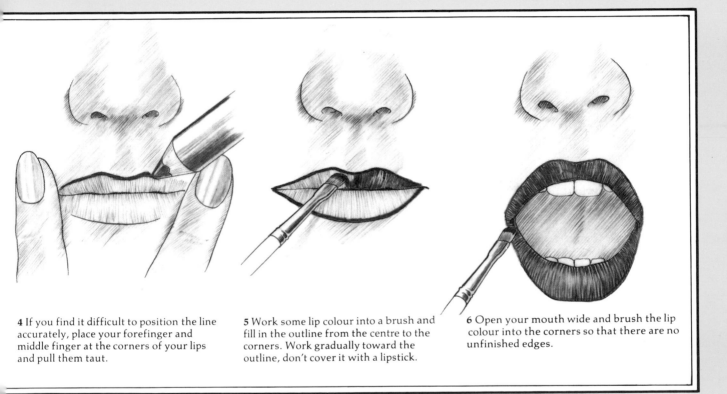

4 If you find it difficult to position the line accurately, place your forefinger and middle finger at the corners of your lips and pull them taut.

5 Work some lip colour into a brush and fill in the outline from the centre to the corners. Work gradually toward the outline, don't cover it with a lipstick.

6 Open your mouth wide and brush the lip colour into the corners so that there are no unfinished edges.

D If only your top or bottom lip lacks fullness, draw your line just outside your natural lip line on the thinner lip. Then fill in the area of the full lip with a darker colour than you use on the thin one.

E To make your lips plumper and more pouting, apply colour over all but the very centre of the lips. Fill in the centre with a lighter, more shimmering colour, but don't make the difference too obvious.

F As you get older, the natural lip line becomes less well defined and is complicated by wrinkle lines running into the lip shape. A hard pencil and a good lipstick coating will help stop the colour seeping beyond the lips themselves. Use gloss sparingly, and choose lipstick colours carefully! If lipstick is too pale it will look washed out, but if it is too bright it will look garish and aging.

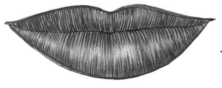

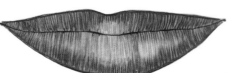

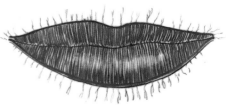

©DIAGRAM

Eye care

The eyes are mirrors of your health and well-being. If you are fit and healthy, eating a nutritious diet, and getting plenty of sleep and exercise, your eyes should be clear, shiny, and slightly moist. If your eyes are red, puffy, bloodshot, or watery, or if they feel strained or gritty, then something is amiss!

TAKING CARE OF YOUR EYES

On the whole, the eyes protect themselves very well. Eyelids close instinctively when dust, smoke, or irritants threaten them, and the pupils contract in bright light. The gentle action of blinking circulates the tears and so keeps the eye clean and clear. Eyelashes catch dust that would otherwise be caught on the eye's moist surface. It is important to make sure that you don't block the tear ducts, as this can easily lead to infection. Around the eyes, the skin is very fine and so is susceptible to damage and dragging. As this skin has no support in the eyesocket from underlying bones, it tends to stretch and wrinkle easily and will be one of the first places to show signs of age.

Use a cream especially designed for use around the eyes. As this is such a delicate area, only the most gentle cream should be applied.

Take good care of your eyes by avoiding so-called eyestrain. Read and do detailed work only in good light, and make sure that your eyes have a rest from these activities every half hour or so. When driving, people tend to blink less often than usual, which can lead to tired eyes; try to remember to blink more frequently. Your eyes will also probably benefit if you try the various activities described below.

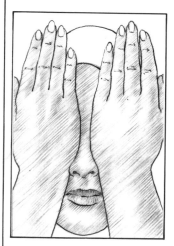

Palming
Place your elbows on a table, close your eyes, and cover them lightly with the palms of your hands. Relax and breathe calmly, and press the outsides of your hands against the cheekbones and browbones for a few minutes (don't press on the eyeballs themselves).

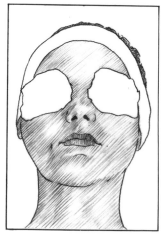

Cold compresses
After the palming exercise cover your eyes with cold compresses made from cotton wool pads dipped in ice-cold tea. Or try some thin slices of chilled cucumber, raw potato, or even iced, used teabags on pads of gauze.

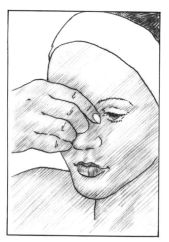

Pinching
Use your thumb and forefinger to press firmly on the sides of your nose at the corner of your eyes, for about 30 seconds. This not only helps to relieve tired eyes, but gets rid of tension and scowl lines.

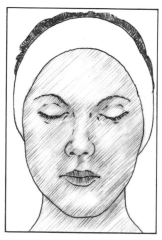

Blinking
Blinking fast helps to wash your eyes when they are dry. Also try closing your eyes extra tightly and then opening them again very slowly; this is a handy way of clearing your vision if it suddenly becomes blurred.

GLASSES

Glasses can be prescribed to correct several common eye defects, particularly short sight, long sight, and astigmatism. Sometimes only one eye is affected, sometimes both; the lenses prescribed will take this into account. Glasses are available in many different styles, so you needn't feel self-conscious about wearing them. Dark glasses with prescription lenses can be obtained for use in strong sunlight, and shatterproof ones for use when playing sport.

CONTACT LENSES

These are alternatives to glasses, and are held in place by the surface tension of the eye's natural lubrication. Contact lenses may be hard or soft. Hard lenses are cheaper than soft ones and are easier to keep clean, but many people have difficulty in accustoming their eyes to wearing them. Soft lenses are easier to adjust to and can generally be worn for longer periods, but they are more expensive and have a shorter life.

COMMON EYE COMPLAINTS

The eyes are prone to a variety of generally minor but sometimes more troublesome problems.

Bloodshot eyes may be caused by smoke or by swimming in chlorinated or salt water, or they may be a symptom of a cold or hayfever. Cold compresses may help.

Sticky eyes are usually caused by conjunctivitis. This infection makes the eye's natural lubrication too thick to be cleared away easily by the tears, and so more dirt is trapped and the eye feels sticky. Consult a doctor immediately, and make sure your towels and facecloths are kept separate from everybody else's, as conjunctivitis spreads very easily.

Red-rimmed eyes may be caused by an infection of the eyelash follicles known as blepharitis. This may be part of a general dermatitis (skin infection) affecting the scalp and ears; see a doctor to obtain a cream to clear up the condition.

Sties are small boils that occur at the root of an eyelash. They start as a small red tender area and develop into an extremely painful pustule. Pull out the affected eyelash with tweezers and bathe your eye with cotton wool dipped in hot water to relieve the pain and bring the sty to a head, but be careful not to allow the pus to spread to other eyelash follicles.

Tired eyes may result from lack of sleep, or from not resting your eyes sufficiently – for instance you may have been staring for too long at a book, a VDU, a motorway, or a stretch of water. Try exercising your eyes with rapid blinking. Eyedrops may help in some cases, although some doctors advise against them.

Foreign bodies in the eye feel very uncomfortable even if they are only specks of dust. Any extraneous object should be removed immediately, before it has a chance to set up an infection; try removing the speck by pulling your upper eyelid over the lower one. If this fails, make a very weak saline solution with one teaspoon of salt in a pint of cooled, boiled water and bathe your eye in this.

Removing a foreign body
1 Pulling the upper lid over the lower one
2 Bathing the eye with a weak saline solution

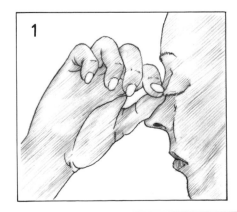
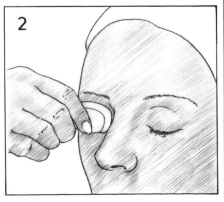

Eye make-up 1

The eyes are usually the most beautiful and expressive part of the face, and skillfully applied make-up will accentuate them. Eye make-up can be very simple – a touch of mascara or a brush of shadow suitable for a busy day or a summer outing. Or it may be very dramatic – several colours of eye-shadow, eyeliner, mascara, and brow pencil for a special night out.

The trick is to learn to apply all your eye cosmetics accurately and skilfully; that you will make every stroke count, whether you need a one-minute miracle in the morning or whether you have 15 minutes to spare before a party. Experiment with different ways of shading and highlighting your eyes, and see which shapes and colours suit you best. Generally, fair complexions look best with softer, more subtle shades of shadow, liner, and mascara, while darker skins can take more dramatic colours and combinations.

USING EYE SHADOW

Eye shadow is the main way of contouring your eyes, and is the most important part of your eye make-up. Always make sure that it is blended well into the surrounding skin or the adjoining colour of shadow; harsh edges will make it look artificial.

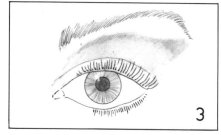

A

Basic rules

Whatever kind of shadow you are using, there are several basic rules to follow.
1 Use neutral tones such as flat browns, greys, grey-greens, and grey-blues to establish the shape of the eye, working from the inner to the outer corner of the eye.
2 Use a darker tone to define the shape of the socket with a contour shadow.
3 Use a lighter tone on the eyelids and beneath the brows to highlight the eyes.

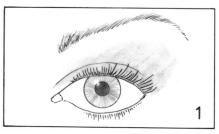

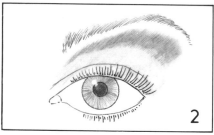

Special techniques

Here are some ways of emphasising your good points and of playing down various slight defects.
A Prominent eyes can be made less obvious by using dark shadow over the whole lid and lighter toner under the brow.
B Deep-set eyes can be brought forward by using pale shadow over the lid and darker shadow on the brow bone.
C Droopy eyes can be given a lift by applying darker shadow in the socket line, stopping it before the droopy corner. Brush your eyebrows upward, and define their shape well with a pencil.
D Sloe-shaped eyes can be emphasised with a deep-toned shadow taken to the outermost part of the lid and extended slightly beyond the corner of the eye. Then apply a light-toned shadow to the inner corner of the eye and extend it to the brow bone.

USING EYELINER

Eyeliner is used to accentuate the shape of your eyes by emphasising the borders of the eyelids and providing a contrast between the dark eyeliner and the white of the eye. It should be applied after your eye shadow.

Eyeliner techniques

1 To apply liquid liner or eyeliner pencil, rest your elbows on a table to steady your hands. Hold the corner of your eye steady with one hand, and with the other gently draw a line just outside your eyelashes on the upper and lower lids.

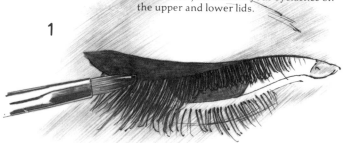

EYE SHADOWS

Eyeshadow is available in various forms; creams, pencils and pressed powder, all with either a matt or pearlised finish. The choice of textures and shades is enormous, allowing you to mix and match and create a variety of different looks.

Powder eyeshadow is the simplest to apply, using either a specially shaped sponge applicator or cosmetic brush. The powder glides on the eyelid and with careful blending you can easily vary the density of colour.

Creams require a little more skill and should be applied with either a brush or fingertip. Powder pencils allow for precise application, while the cream formulations tend to crease in the eyelid.

EYELINERS

Eyeliner comes in three main forms: liquid, and two types of pencil. Liquid is supplied in a small bottle with a fine brush; it needs to be applied carefully so that the line doesn't look too harsh. Some eyeliner pencils are water-soluble; they have to be moistened with water or saliva before being applied and will give either a hard or gentle line as required. Other eyeliner pencils are used without moistening them; before buying this type of pencil, test that it is not too hard by using it on the fine skin between your thumb and first finger and checking that it does not drag or catch the skin.

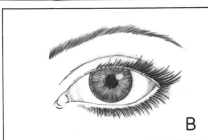

B

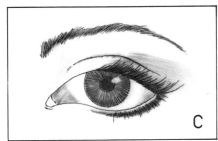

C

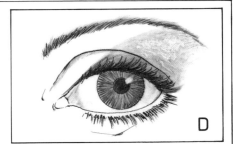

D

E If your eyes are close-set, throw the emphasis to the outer corners by applying a dark-toned shadow to the outer half and extending it slightly beyond the corner of the eye. Then apply a light-toned shadow to the inner half of the eye.

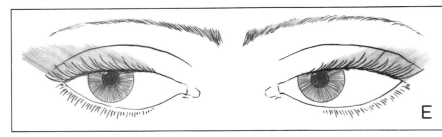

E

F If you have wide-set eyes, accentuate the inner corner. Starting close to your nose, use a darker shadow to cover the inner half of the eye. Shade the outer half of the eye in a lighter tone, and do not extend it past the corner of the eye.

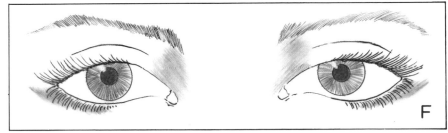

F

2 For a more subtle effect, use an eye pencil in the same colour as your eye shadow but a little darker. Dot the pencil all along your upper lashes and just below the lower ones. Gently blend the eyeshadow into the dots with your fingertip.

3 For a very striking effect, use an eye pencil or kohl pencil to draw a line along the inside of your upper and lower lids, right next to your eye. This can make your eyes look enormous, but if they are fairly small it may make them seem even smaller.

It is best to avoid this technique if your eyes are very sensitive to cosmetics.

2

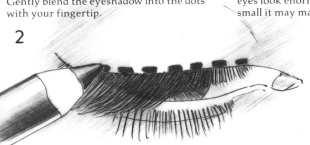

3

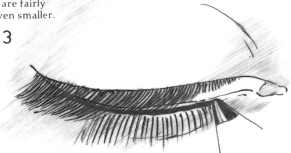

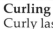

EYELASHES

Emphasising the eyelashes accentuates the eyes in general and adds an attractive finishing touch to your eye make-up.

Mascara

Waterproof and non-waterproof mascaras are available. Non-waterproof ones are best for regular use as they are easier to remove. Waterproof mascaras are useful for swimmers but must always be removed very carefully to avoid damaging the delicate skin around the eyes. The most usual colours for mascara are black, dark brown, and charcoal, although blue and green are also available.

Applying mascara
As shown below, close one eye and brush mascara down from the roots to the tips of your lashes. Next, open your eye wide and brush the top lashes from underneath, again from roots to tips. Then, again with your eye open and working from roots to tips, add more mascara to the lower lashes. Repeat for the other eye.

Curling

Curly lashes look thicker and so need less mascara. Straight lashes can be curled with eyelash curlers; carefully trap a row of lashes in the curlers and apply several short squeezes.

Dyeing

The eyelashes can be dyed cosmetically to make them more apparent. Eyelash dyeing is quite difficult to do, so you will probably be better to get this job done professionally rather than trying to do it yourself. Avoid dark dyes if your natural lash colour is very pale.

False eyelashes

These can be worn to give very different effects: they can look very obvious, or they can be trimmed back to different lengths to be more discreet and natural looking. False eyelashes are attached with a special glue, but because this is not particularly easy to remove completely it is advisable not to wear false eyelashes very frequently.

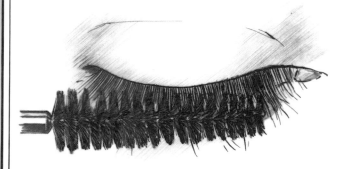

REMOVING EYE MAKE-UP

All eye make-up must be thoroughly removed if left-over traces are not to dry out and damage the delicate tissue that surrounds the eyes. Mascara in particular is very easy to miss; after your regular eye make-up cleansing procedure, try removing final traces of mascara with a cotton-tipped stick dipped in cleanser.

Cleansing procedure
Begin by applying eye make-up remover directly to a cotton wool pad. With your eye closed, draw the pad over the upper lid, starting from the inside corner of the eye. Again with your eye closed, use the other side of the pad for the lower lid. Continue with a clean pad until no more make-up can be removed. Then repeat this procedure for the other eye, always using a different pad. Finish off by gently patting the eyes with a tissue to remove any surplus cleansing cream.

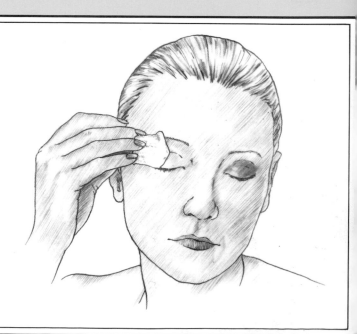

EYEBROWS

The eyebrows are an important part of your overall face shape and expression, and should not be neglected when you are thinking of eye make-up. If your eyebrows are in good shape they will balance the features and provide a frame for your eyes. If the eyebrows are very thin and hard they will look unnatural: if they are very thick and shaggy they will tend to look unfeminine and to overshadow your eyes.

Shaping

The natural shape of your eyebrows and the place on the brow where they grow will probably be a natural balance to your face shape. This means that it is usually best not to alter their shape too drastically. A good way of establishing where your eyebrows should begin and end and how high they should arch is to use the simple measuring technique shown on this page. If you have a small brow and fine features, your eyebrows should be delicate too. If your features are heavy, then your eyebrows may need strengthening and defining more clearly if they are to play their full part.

Plucking

Removing straggling hairs from around the edges of your eyebrows and also removing any very bushy hairs will improve the outline of your eyebrows. But take care not to remove too many hairs or your eyebrows may end up looking rather bald and unnatural. It is a good idea to pluck your eyebrows after taking a hot bath, as the skin is softer then and the hair follicles are more open. You will probably find that slant-ended tweezers are better for plucking the eyebrows than either straight- or round-ended ones; use the technique illustrated on this page. After plucking your eyebrows, give them another brushing with your eyebrow brush, and then wipe them with a mild toner to close the follicles that have had their hairs removed.

Defining

Most people prefer to use a fine eyebrow pencil for defining their eyebrows. Always choose a colour to tone with your own eyebrows and hair colour: your face will look strange if you choose a colour that is at odds with your natural colouring. If you are using an eyebrow pencil make sure that it is very sharp so that you can draw the lines exactly where you want them. Use a brush to rid your eyebrows of any foundation or face powder and then use the technique shown on this page.

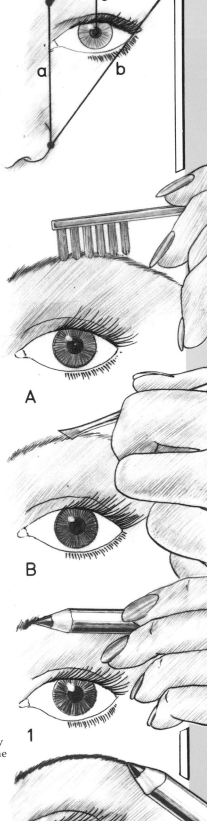

Measuring the eyebrows
Sit in front of a mirror and take a pencil in one hand.
a Hold the pencil so that it makes a line from the side of your nostril to the inner corner of your eye and upward: where the pencil touches the eyebrow is where your eyebrow should start.
b Hold the pencil at an angle from the side of the nostril, past the outer corner of your eye and outward: this is where your eyebrow should end.
c If you look straight ahead, the highest point of your eyebrow should be directly above the iris of your eye.

Plucking the eyebrows
A First brush your eyebrows into shape with a special eyebrow brush or a clean old toothbrush.
B Then use tweezers to pluck out the stray hairs. Begin by removing stragglers from between your eyebrows and then tidy up the general outline.

Defining the eyebrows
1 Always start at the inner corner of the eyebrow and use short, light upward strokes as you work toward the middle.
2 From the centre of the eyebrow to the outer edge, use the same kind of feathery strokes as before but this time tip them downward.

Your teeth and gums are very important to the overall effect of your face; you show them when you talk, smile, laugh, or even yawn! Two rows of clean, white, well cared for teeth in healthy pink gums are an asset to any face, and it's worth taking the time to keep them in peak condition.

CLEANING YOUR TEETH

Cleaning your teeth by brushing and flossing benefits them in several ways. First of all it makes them look more attractive by removing food particles and plaque – the sticky, yellowish film that clings to uncleaned teeth. Removing the plaque regularly should also keep dental caries – tooth decay – to a minimum; the longer plaque remains on the teeth, the more chance it has to eat into the enamel. Thorough cleaning also helps to keep your breath fresh, and your gums in good condition. The blood supply to the gums is stimulated by the brushing, and plaque is removed before it has a chance to creep under the gums and cause problems.

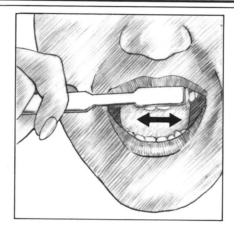

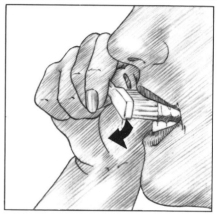

Brushing technique
1 Apply toothpaste to your brush and then place the brush against your teeth as shown. Then brush, moving the brush slightly from side to side so that the bristles reach into the gap between your teeth and gums.

2 Starting with the brush at the junction of your teeth and gums, brush away from the gums with an outward rotating movement. Repeat steps 1 and 2 until you have cleaned the outsides of all your upper and lower teeth.

CARING FOR YOUR TEETH

Teeth should be brushed after every meal, as plaque can form in only a few hours. Foods that are sweet, such as sweets and soft drinks, or starchy, such as cakes and potatoes, cling to the teeth and form plaque very quickly. If you must eat between meals, eat fruit or nuts or raw vegetables to keep your teeth as plaque-free as possible. Crisp vegetables such as raw carrot or celery actually help to clean the teeth. Cut down on sweetened tea, coffee, or chocolate drinks; these are just as bad for your teeth as sweets. Also avoid constantly chewing sweetened gum, as this bathes the mouth in sugar and can spell disaster for your teeth.

It is important to seek regular professional dental care even if you maintain a good cleaning routine and a healthy diet; with the best will in the world you may occasionally need a filling or a professional clean and polish. Visit your dentist at least twice a year so that he or she can arrest any problems before they become serious, and can also give you any oral hygiene advice. Your dentist may apply a fissure sealant or fluoride to your teeth to help prevent decay, but don't rely on these and neglect your own cleaning routine. Occasionally your teeth may be unexpectedly damaged. Avoid accidents to your teeth as much as possible: wear a gumshield if you are involved in potentially damaging sports, and never open bottles or crack nuts with your teeth. If you do chip a tooth or lose a filling or a crown, see your dentist quickly, before decay sets in. If a whole tooth is knocked out, rinse it in clean water and replace it in its socket and then rush to the hospital or to a dentist; it may be possible for them to splint the tooth so that it will reestablish itself in the gum.

TOOTHBRUSHES AND TOOTHPASTES

It is important to choose a good toothbrush so that you can get the maximum benefit from it. Avoid brushes that are very hard; although it may seem that they give your teeth a really good clean, they may damage the tender gums. On the other hand, a toothbrush that is too soft will not brush plaque away effectively. Synthetic fibres are better than natural bristle, as bristle tends to harbour germs more easily. Change your toothbrush regularly, as soon as the bristles start to splay. Toothpaste is, literally, very much a matter of taste. Some formulas contain fluoride, which is recommended by many dental associations; others contain extra ingredients for freshening the breath.

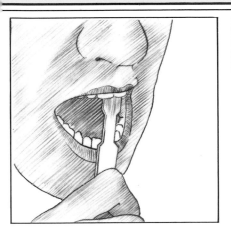

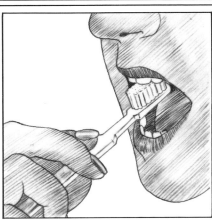

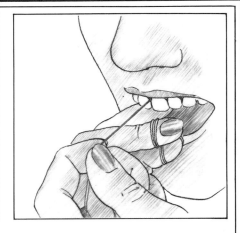

3 Next brush to and fro across the biting and chewing surfaces of your teeth, making sure that you reach right to the very back.

4 Finally brush the insides of your teeth; the best way of brushing the insides of your front teeth is to hold the brush in an almost vertical position, as illustrated, and then brush up or down away from the gums.

5 At least once a day, use dental floss to finish off your teeth cleaning routine. Wind a length of floss around the second finger of each hand, leaving about 2 inches of floss between them. Then move the floss gently up and down between your teeth.

BACK-UP EQUIPMENT

In addition to your regular toothbrush, toothpaste, and dental floss, all of which are available in a considerable variety of types and sizes, it is possible to buy a number of other dental hygiene items that will help you maintain a really thorough teeth care routine.

An interdental brush has a small head set at an angle to the handle; this makes it easier to clean the crevices between the teeth and also to brush the very back teeth more thoroughly.

Tooth polishes can be used to give your teeth an extra-clean feel or to remove occasional stains. But don't make frequent use of abrasive polishes as these can damage your tooth enamel.

Wooden toothpicks can be very useful for a quick clean between the teeth. Most toothpicks are triangular in shape; place one flat side against your gum and then move the point of the triangle between your teeth.

Disclosing tablets are useful for revealing any parts of your teeth that you are failing to reach during your regular brushing routine. After cleaning your teeth, dissolve a disclosing tablet in water and rinse your mouth with the solution; any plaque that you have failed to brush away will now be stained and clearly visible. (Don't try the disclosing tablet test just before you are intending to go out!)

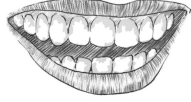

Disclosing tablet test
As shown here, disclosing tablets make it very easy to see plaque on the teeth.

Even if you follow a very thorough tooth care routine, the time will probably come when your teeth or gums need professional intervention. Ideally you should visit your dentist every six months: if anything does go wrong with your teeth it can then be put right as quickly as possible so that the damage is minimised. As well as helping you keep your mouth healthy, your dentist will also be able to advise you on the latest developments in cosmetic dentistry.

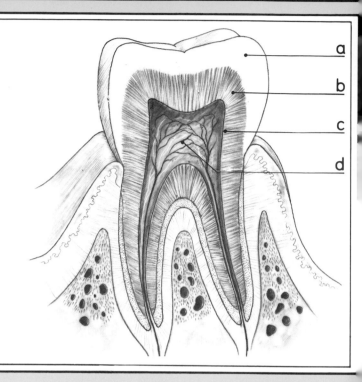

Structure of the teeth
Teeth consist of a hard outer shell and a soft core; the core contains pulp, nerves, and blood vessels. The part of the tooth jutting from the jaw is called the crown; the root is the part embedded in the jaw.

a Enamel forms the hard outside surface of the tooth.
b Dentine is slightly softer than enamel and forms the bulk of the tooth.
c Cementum is a hard coating on the root of the tooth.
d Pulp is a soft body tissue.

VENEER CAPPING

Veneer capping is an alternative to the traditional porcelain cap for an unsightly or damaged tooth – provided that the tooth itself is healthy. The veneer is a thin slice of acrylic laminate, about the thickness of a fingernail, that is bonded into place over the tooth to be repaired.

Compared with traditional crowning or capping, veneer capping is quick, economical, and painless. The tooth remains whole under the veneer and, being sealed, does not decay. If the veneer is removed, the tooth will remineralise itself. Veneer caps will last for several years and can be replaced without problems when necessary.

Unfortunately, veneer capping is not suitable for all unsightly teeth. It cannot be used on molars, where the constant grinding and chewing action would damage the laminate. Very badly broken teeth can only be veneer capped if enough tooth surface remains for a good bond to be formed.

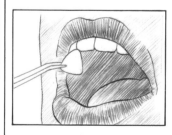
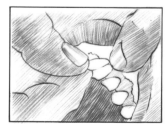
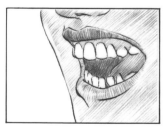
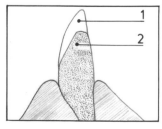

1 A piece of veneer of the correct size and colour to match the other teeth is carefully chosen. To prepare the tooth to take the veneer, the dentist cleans off any stains and then roughens the surface of the tooth enamel with a weak acid solution. The tooth is then painted with sealant.

2 The veneer is painted with bonding material and then carefully put into place, extending up just under the gum. The bonding material grips easily onto the roughened surface of the tooth. A 20 second burst of ultraviolet light is used to set the bond.

3 The veneer is buffed and polished to match the shape and appearance of the other teeth in the mouth.

Paste capping
An alternative to veneer capping is paste capping. A paste (**1**) made of plastic, finely ground quartz, glass, or silica, is applied to the cleaned and etched tooth (**2**) and sculpted into shape by the dentist.

PROBLEMS AND TREATMENTS

Discolouration Some drugs taken in childhood can cause discolouration of the permanent teeth, but the most common causes of tooth staining are smoking, or a high consumption of tea, coffee, or red wine. A thick discolouring film on the teeth is a build-up of plaque. Professional scaling and polishing will deal with most stains; stains that do not respond to this treatment can be hidden by veneer caps.

Cavities These begin when plaque eats into the surface of the tooth's enamel. As the decay eats deeper into the dentine, a dark cavity appears, and the tooth becomes sensitive and then painful when the pulp is reached. The dentist drills out all the decayed matter, then packs the cleaned cavity with a suitable filling. This may be amalgam (a metal compound that looks silvery when it hardens), gold, or one of the newer "white fillings" that match your teeth and so look less unsightly. The white fillings are not as strong as the metal fillings, and so some dentists are only willing to use them to fill small cavities. The sooner any cavity is treated, the better.

Broken teeth Various professional treatments are available to improve teeth that are chipped, broken, or worn into ridges. Veneering is the quickest and simplest way to deal with the problem, but a badly damaged tooth may need a traditional crown or cap. The tooth is filed down to a peg, and then an artificial cap or crown is cemented onto it to build up the shape of the tooth again. Even a tooth that has been broken off near the gum can be treated in this way if an artificial support peg is inserted. The caps can be made of various materials, including porcelain and plastics, and the colour can be matched to the existing teeth. At the back of the mouth, where strength is usually more important than appearance, caps are usually made of gold or alloy. A well-fitting cap should be a permanent fixture.

Missing teeth Various types of bridges can be used to fit artificial teeth into the gaps left by extractions or when a tooth has been knocked out accidentally. They may be made of gold, gold and porcelain, or plastic. Some bridges can be attached to the adjacent teeth with small metal wires or wings that are then bonded into place; other types can only be anchored into place by crowning or capping the adjacent teeth. The exact type of bridge chosen will depend on the size of the gap and the number of teeth missing.

If you are unfortunate enough to lose more than just one or two of your teeth, you may need a partial or a full set of false teeth or dentures. These are usually made of plastic and are carefully shaped to fit well over your gums and palate. Partial dentures usually need to be held in place among your real teeth by clasps or brackets; complete sets of false teeth should fit well enough not to need supports or adhesives. All dentures must be removed every day for thorough cleaning.

Implants are an alternative to bridges or dentures. They are false teeth permanently anchored in the jawbone by means of a metal pin. Cosmetically they are probably preferable to false teeth, but they carry the risk of the gum rejecting the artificial materials or becoming infected. Implants usually have to be replaced after about five years.

Crooked teeth There are many ways of straightening crooked or buck teeth, but treatment should ideally begin before adolescence. For older people, straightening may mean considering extensive orthodontic surgery.

Gingevitis This is inflammation of the gums caused by a build-up of plaque around the gum margins. The gums can become swollen, red, and tender, and liable to bleed when the teeth are cleaned. Professional removal of the plaque build-up is necessary.

Peridontal pockets These are gaps between the gums and the teeth that occur when plaque is allowed to build up and force its way under the gums. As the pocket enlarges, the fibrous attachments holding the teeth in place weaken, and the teeth may eventually loosen and fall out. The pockets can be cut back: the loosened outer margin of the gum is sliced away and the gum allowed to heal. If the teeth are kept perfectly clean the problem should not recur.

A peridontal abscess is an infection that can occur in a peridontal pocket when food debris has lodged there and decayed. Abscesses need to be drained immediately to relieve the pain and remove the source of infection.

Ear care

With a little basic care your ears should remain trouble-free for most of your life. The main thing to remember is that the ears are usually very efficient organs and have their own self-cleansing mechanism. The less they are interfered with, the healthier they will be.

CLEANING YOUR EARS

You need a certain amount of wax in your ears. The wax attracts dirt and potential irritants as they enter the ear and stops them from travelling farther down the ear canal. It also keeps the ear moist, supple, and slightly insulated. If you remove all the wax you are removing your ears' defence mechanism. Gently clean your ears daily with a warm washcloth over a finger. Trying to clean the ears out farther with cotton tipped buds, bobby pins, etc, will only force wax down into the ear canal and may damage the ear's delicate lining. If your ears do become blocked with wax, ask your doctor to syringe them – a simple process which uses warm water to ease the plug of wax free. Do not attempt to remove the wax plug yourself.

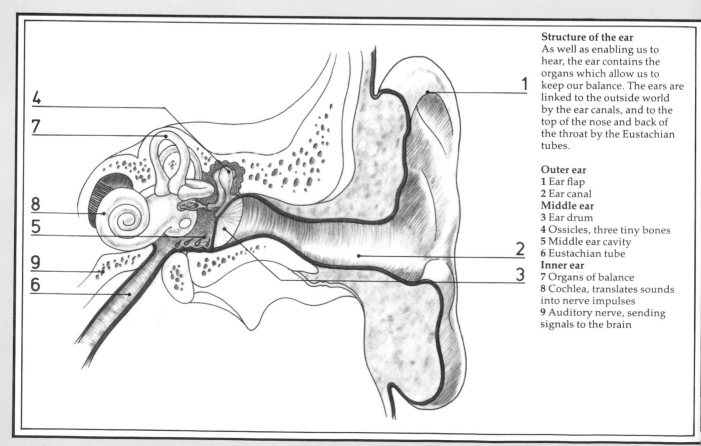

Structure of the ear
As well as enabling us to hear, the ear contains the organs which allow us to keep our balance. The ears are linked to the outside world by the ear canals, and to the top of the nose and back of the throat by the Eustachian tubes.

Outer ear
1 Ear flap
2 Ear canal
Middle ear
3 Ear drum
4 Ossicles, three tiny bones
5 Middle ear cavity
6 Eustachian tube
Inner ear
7 Organs of balance
8 Cochlea, translates sounds into nerve impulses
9 Auditory nerve, sending signals to the brain

AVOIDING EAR DAMAGE

Noise can cause permanent ear damage. If you are exposed to a high level of noise at work, wear industrial earmuffs for protection. Avoid noisy discos and concerts, and keep the volume of music on your personal stereo down to a safe level. Water in the ear can also cause complications. If you go swimming, it is very important to protect your ears: wearing a swim cap or waterproof earplugs will help. Dry your ears carefully with a soft towel when you come out of the water, and if water is trapped in one ear lie on that side until the water runs out. This will help you avoid "swimmer's ear" – an infection of the outer ear that occurs in moist conditions.

The ears are very sensitive to pressure changes of all kinds. Some people notice this when they are travelling in aeroplanes or lifts, when they feel as if their ears are blocked. This feeling can often be relieved by yawning, swallowing, or sucking sweets. Other people feel discomfort in their ears when they are swimming underwater. Try taking a deep breath before you submerge and hold it when you are underwater: this should help to equalise the pressure in your ears. If you go scuba diving, pay particular attention to the drill for relieving pressure in your ears.

EAR PROBLEMS

Earache is often caused by an infection of the middle ear. It may occur in conjunction with a nose or throat infection, as the germs can travel up the Eustachian tube. The ear is painful because the pressure behind the eardrum has been altered. Consult your doctor if the earache is severe. Discharges from the ear are not natural, and you should always consult your doctor if your ear is producing a watery, bloodstained, or infected discharge. A discharge may be a sign that something is stuck in the ear canal, or that there is an infection deeper in the ear. Ear infections should always be taken seriously. Inner ear infections can cause vomiting, deafness, and loss of balance. If the condition is not treated rapidly the deafness and disturbed balance may become permanent.

Boils inside the ear are bacterial infections that can be caused by scratching the ear canal, perhaps with a dirty fingernail. They can be intensely painful. Holding a warm compress to the ear may help to relieve the pain temporarily, and your doctor will be able to advise you how to deal with the infection.

Loss of hearing can be caused by damage to the eardrum, damage to the auditory nerves after some severe illnesses, or as part of the aging process. If you suffer any loss of hearing, you should seek professional advice immediately. You should also seek advice if you suffer from tinnitus – a ringing or other constant sound in the ears, that may be temporary or permanent.

Ear piercing

If you enjoy wearing earrings you may well decide to have your ears pierced one or more times. This is a perfectly safe procedure providing that it is carried out under sterile conditions. The high speed piercing guns commonly used these days are safe and sterile in professional hands. The operator will clean the lobes of your ears with spirit or alcohol, and will then mark them with the position for the studs. Check these marks carefully: you cannot change your mind about their position after your ears have been pierced! The gun will then be used to fire a sterile stud into your earlobe. You will be advised to keep the studs in your ears for about six weeks, turning them regularly, and keeping the area around them clean with spirit. Once the holes are completely healed you can remove the studs and replace them with your own earrings. If you insert your earrings with dirty hands or leave them in too long you may infect your ears. Remove your earrings at least once a day and clean your lobes thoroughly. Avoid allergic reactions by ensuring that your earrings have gold, silver, or hypoallergenic shafts or wires, and by not securing the metal butterflies too tightly.

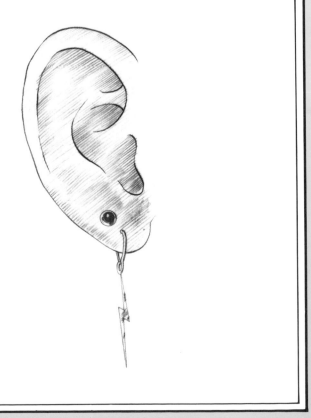

Cosmetic surgery

Cosmetic surgery can be used to correct a real or imagined defect (for instance operations to reshape the nose or to pin back the ears), or to eradicate some of the signs of aging, particularly wrinkles and sagging muscles.

The operations can sound deceptively simple, but it is never a light undertaking to submit yourself to anaesthetic, stitches, bruising, convalescence, and the risk of possible infection. Operations of any sort should always be taken seriously, and if you are considering cosmetic surgery it is worth asking yourself a few honest questions before you go ahead.

Why do I want the operation – honestly? The border between a necessary correction and pure vanity can be hard to determine; only you know your true motives.

Do I have a realistic expectation of what the operation will do for me? It is no use hoping that removing wrinkles will improve basic personality problems, or that a new nose shape will turn you into a film-star beauty overnight.

Can the results I want, or some of them, be achieved in any other way? Maybe there are tricks with make-up, hairstyle, or fashion that will save the expense and the risk of surgery.

FACE LIFTS

A face lift does not aim to get rid of all the lines in a woman's face: the art lies in giving just enough lift to leave the natural expression lines, while eradicating the worst signs of age and stress. Incisions are made parallel to the edges of the scalp, about three quarters of an inch into the hairline so that the scar will not show. During the face lift, excess skin and fat are removed, and the underlying muscles and tissues are pulled back at right angles to the incision. Face lift operations take about two hours. They cause a great deal of swelling and bruising of the face, but this soon begins to subside. The stitches in the hairline are removed after about two weeks. The best results are seen about six months after the operation, after the face has had time to settle down again. The effects of a face lift operation generally last for about six years.

Three of the most popular face lift operations are described here.

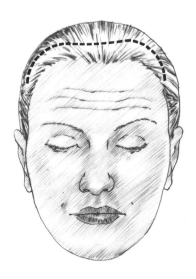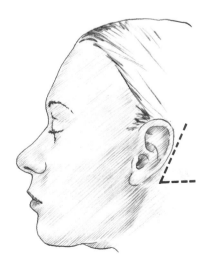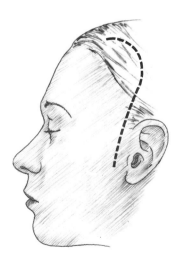

The brow lift
This aims to smooth out worry lines and wrinkles across the brow. The cut is made across the top of the hairline, and the skin is pulled up and back.

The jawline lift
This aims to get rid of sagging jowls and to make the jawline firmer. The incision is made behind the ears and down behind the hairline away from the chin.

The mini lift
This aims to tighten sagging skin around the middle of the face. The incision runs inside the hairline and then in front of the ears, where it is hidden by a fold of skin.

SURGERY INVOLVING SPECIFIC FEATURES

The overall appearance of a person's face can sometimes be changed quite considerably by surgery involving a particular feature. Most common are operations involving the eyelids, nose, chin, or ears.

Eyelid surgery

Eyelid surgery, or blepharoplasty, can remove drooping skin from the eyelids, change the shape of the eyelids or brow, or get rid of bags under the eyes. Surgery is typically straightforward and may be carried out on an outpatient basis. The stitches are removed after only two or three days. Healing is rapid and scarring is usually slight. Initial swelling and bruising may take a couple of weeks to subside, but dark glasses can be worn to conceal them.

Nose surgery

Surgical reshaping of the nose, or rhinoplasty, is one of the commonest and most successful of all cosmetic operations. A crooked nose can be straightened, a large nose made smaller, or a small one made larger. Operations are performed from inside the nose so there is no visible scarring. To reduce the size of the nose, the surgeon cuts out excess bone and cartilage. To remodel or increase the size of the nose, implants of cartilage or silicone can be made. A hospital stay of three to four days is usually necessary.

Chin surgery

Operations can make the chin smaller or larger. A protruding chin can be reduced by removing some of the bone, or a small or receding chin can be built up by the insertion of a molded plastic implant. Chin operations involve a general anaesthetic and a short hospital stay. A tight bandage must be worn for about 10 days after an implant operation.

Ear surgery

Cosmetic surgery on the ears, or otoplasty, will permanently "pin back" protruding ears. In adults the operation is generally carried out under a local anaesthetic on an outpatient basis. A dressing must be worn around the head for at least one week.

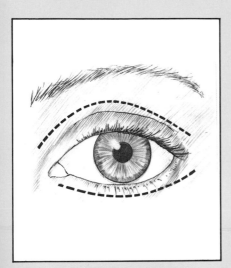

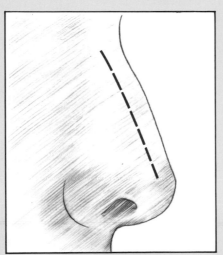

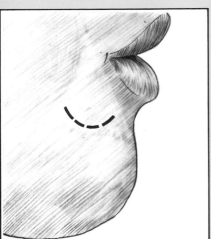

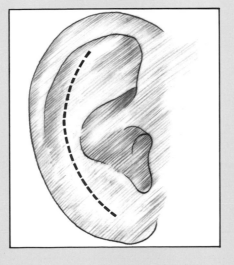

Eyelid surgery
Incisions are made in the hollow under the brow bone, or just below the lashes of the lower lid.

Nose surgery
The surgeon makes the incision inside the nose to avoid external scarring.

Chin surgery
This involves either an incision from inside the mouth, along the gum line, or an external incision below the chin.

Ear surgery
Excess cartilage is removed through an incision made just behind the ear.

Chapter 4

your hair

Having beautiful, shiny, healthy hair makes you feel wonderful. It is the great confidence builder and morale booster – just washing your hair can lift your spirits, and a new hair style that suits you perfectly can make all the difference to the way that you see yourself. Work at keeping your hair in the peak of condition, and then take advantage of its infinite adaptability to change the style, colour, and cut as often as you like.

Hair growth and types

Correct care is important if you want your hair to look at its best all the time. Get to know your hair – what is your hair type? What length and styles of hair cut suit you best? Can you enhance your hair with colours, conditioners, sets, perms, hairpieces, or wigs? Even the type of brush and comb that you use can be important. If you care for it well, your hair can reflect your personality and enhance your total appearance.

HAIR STRUCTURE

Although hair grows, the hair that we see is technically dead; growth comes from the hair follicle, under the surface of the scalp, that pushes the main hair shaft farther out. The hair shaft is composed mainly of keratin – the same substance that forms fingernails and toenails. Each hair has a spongy core or medulla, covered with a stronger layer called the cortex. The outside of the hair is covered with overlapping scales of keratin. When the hair is in good condition, the keratin scales will be shiny and lie flat; if your hair is tangled, dry, or damaged, the scales will be ruffled, which will give your hair a dull appearance and a rough texture..

Structure of the hair
1 Hair shaft
2 Hair root
3 Follicle
4 Papilla, the growth point
5 Medulla
6 Cortex
7 Cuticle
8 Sebaceous gland

HAIR GROWTH

Most people have 100,000–200,000 hairs on their head. Redheads, although they have the thickest hairs, generally have the fewest number of individual strands. Brunettes have more hairs, while blonds, even though their hair is generally fine in texture, tend to have the most strands. Hair does not grow at a constant rate; it grows faster in hot weather than in cold, for example. On average it will grow about half an inch per month. The growth phase for each hair varies from person to person; the average is about 3–5 years. At the end of the growth phase the follicle enters a resting phase. The old hair remains in the follicle during this phase and is known as a club hair because of its clubbed end. When the growth phase begins again the club hair is pushed out by the new hair growing underneath. On average you lose up to 100 club hairs each day, but as the growth and resting phases are distributed evenly among the hairs on the scalp, you do not notice any obvious patches of hair loss.
Various illnesses and general poor health can

affect the hair's growth, as well as its condition. Some people find it difficult to grow their hair long, while others find it very easy. This is the result of your particular combination of growth rate and hair life-span; only if your hair has a fast growth rate and a long life-span can you quickly and successfully grow your hair long.
The total number of hairs decreases as we get older. After the age of about 30 the process of cell division slows down, so that some hairs drop out and are not replaced. The rate at which you lose your hair is determined genetically, and the process cannot be halted; hair loss happens more often (and more quickly) to men than to women. Grey hair occurs when the hairs are formed without their natural pigmentation; again, nothing can be done to halt this process, although the results can be disguised! Some people start to develop grey hairs in their twenties; others may take another 20 or 30 years before they have a significant number.

HAIR TYPE

Your hair type is relevant to every aspect of hair care, from shampooing and blow drying to cutting and perming.

Hair condition is the first consideration: this will affect the kind of hair-care products you choose, how often you wash your hair, and whether your hair can be permed or coloured.

Oily hair generally goes with oily skin; overactive sebaceous glands in the scalp coat the hair with excess sebum, which makes it lank and lifeless. The grease attracts dust, so the hair needs frequent washing. Hair may become more oily during times of illness or stress; it also can alter with your hormonal level, for instance during the premenstrual phase. Oily hair is often less of a problem during the last six months of pregnancy.

Dry hair occurs when the sebaceous glands produce too little sebum to keep the surface of the hair supple and shiny. This may be caused artificially, if the hair has been damaged by overexposure to sunlight, too much perming, or too-frequent washing. Dry hair looks dull and feels brittle; it often splits easily at the ends, and loses elasticity. Dry hair has little natural protection, and so needs extra protection against hot sunshine, over-hot hairdryers, chlorinated water, and seawater.

Normal hair is shiny and healthy, usually a result of good general health and careful management.

Combination hair is oily at the scalp and roots while the ends of the hairs are dry and frizzy. This can happen to sufferers from dandruff, as the oil soaks into the dry flakes on the scalp instead of travelling along the hair shaft; it may also happen to oily hair when it grows long and the ends become damaged.

Hair texture Are your individual hairs fine, thick, coarse, curly, frizzy, flyaway, straight, wavy? Your hair's texture will affect its care and conditioning, and also the styles that will suit you best.

Hair thickness is particularly relevant to hairstyle. Is your head of hair very fine and wispy, or thick and luxuriant – or somewhere in between?

Hair colour is an important consideration if you are thinking about tints, highlights, bleaching, etc. For instance, if your hair is very dark, it will look unnatural if it is bleached – and the amount of chemical necessary will probably damage it. If it has reddish tints these can be emphasised or played down. If your hair is very fair you probably have a very pale pink complexion – in this case your face would be overwhelmed if you were to dye your hair a dark colour.

Hair and health Your hair is a barometer of your general health; if your body is unfit and undernourished your hair will look dull and lifeless. Your diet should include yeast, or yeast extracts, offal, wholegrains, and eggs – these are all rich in the vitamin B complex thought to play a crucial role in the hair's health. Get plenty of sleep, as during sleep blood is diverted to the scalp and helps to supply nutrients to the follicles; scalp massage can also have the same effect (see p. 153). Exercise, too, is important for healthy hair as well as for good skin and general fitness.

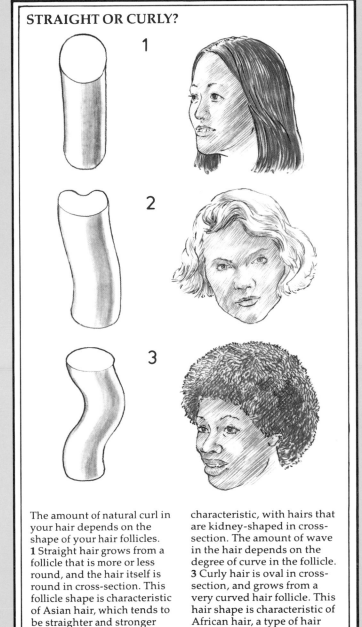

STRAIGHT OR CURLY?

The amount of natural curl in your hair depends on the shape of your hair follicles.
1 Straight hair grows from a follicle that is more or less round, and the hair itself is round in cross-section. This follicle shape is characteristic of Asian hair, which tends to be straighter and stronger than Caucasian hair.
2 Wavy hair is a Caucasian characteristic, with hairs that are kidney-shaped in cross-section. The amount of wave in the hair depends on the degree of curve in the follicle.
3 Curly hair is oval in cross-section, and grows from a very curved hair follicle. This hair shape is characteristic of African hair, a type of hair that tends as well to be very delicate and easily damaged.

©DIAGRAM

Hair care equipment

You will find it much easier to care for your hair properly if you have the right equipment. The right tool for a particular stage of hair care will save time and be more efficient. The equipment need not be expensive, either; the secret is in selecting a tool to do the task properly, so that you are not always making do with second-best. Cleanliness is very important with all hair equipment – it's no use keeping your hair clean if you then use a dirty brush or wrap it round dirty rollers. Brushes and combs should be cleaned of loose hairs after every use, and washed out with shampoo and warm water every time you wash your hair. Rollers and pins, too, can benefit from occasional water treatments. Never use anyone else's combs, brushes, or rollers; in the interests of hygiene keep your hair-care equipment to yourself.

Combs are staple hair-care equipment. Wide-tooth combs are useful for disentangling hair, and for combing conditioner through wet or damp hair. Styling or cutting combs have teeth that are closer together – some have widely-spaced teeth at one end and closer ones at the other. These combs are made of plastic or metal, and are used for styling and for holding hair in position while it is cut. Rattail combs are generally made of metal and are used for making careful divisions of the hair when cutting or styling. Long-tooth or afro combs are used for very curly or thick hair; they lift the hair away from the roots rather than smoothing it.

Brushes should be chosen carefully; make sure that they do not have any rough bristles that will split or damage the hair. Rubber-cushioned brushes or quill brushes with well-spaced plastic bristles are best for use on wet hair. Hair is very easily stretched and damaged when wet, so the bristles should be smooth and not too close together. Natural bristle or bristle-mix brushes have splayed bunches of bristles that are good for brushing through short, wavy, or curly hair, and that can be used to style hair that is slightly damp. Round styling brushes generally have natural bristles all the way round, and are used for shaping styles when blow-drying.

Clips of various shapes are used to hold wet hair in position so that it dries in curls or waves or in a specific direction. Some pins are also used to hold particular styles in place invisibly. Large hairpins are used for anchoring rollers once the hair has been wound round; metal clips are used to make single pincurls, or to hold bangs in position as they dry. Grips and fine hairpins are used for making pincurls, and for securing finished styles such as topknots, French pleats, and chignons; they can be bought in various shades to match different hair colours.

1 Wide-tooth comb
2 Styling comb
3 Rattail comb
4 Long-tooth comb

5 Quill brush
6 Bristle hairbrush
7 Round styling brush

8 Large hairgrips
9 Metal clips
10 Hairgrips
11 Fine hairpins

148

Rollers or curlers are used on damp hair; they hold it in position while it dries so that it is shaped into curls or waves. Spiky rollers should be used carefully or they can tear the hair. With foam rollers the hair is wound round and secured with a plastic bar and a pin; when the hair is dry it forms into soft curls. Mesh rollers are used a great deal in the hairstyling profession; they are held in place with clips and give a tight curl.

Styling wands or tongs are generally used to curl individual strands of hair. The strand is held in place under a loose bar and wound around the heated wand. The longer it is held on the wand, the tighter the curl. Styling wands can also be used to straighten curly hair temporarily.

Heated styling brushes have short bristles to hold the hair in place, and are powered by electricity or by small gas cylinders. The hair is wound round the bristles and the heat sets it into curls.

Heated rollers are warmed by an electric current and then positioned in dry hair; they give a quick, short-term set or a boost to a drooping hairstyle.

Hairdriers are used to speed up the natural drying process. Drying needs to be done very carefully; if too much heat is applied, or if the drier is too close to the scalp, the hair can be damaged or the scalp burned. Dry hair is especially sensitive to over-vigorous drying, and too much heat strips it of still more of its protective coating.

Blow-driers are the most commonly used home drying equipment. They are available in many different designs; some have combs and brushes that can be attached for achieving specific styles, others end in a nozzle that can be directed very accurately at particular portions of the hair. All good driers will have variable heat settings and an automatic cutout system in case the power supply is overloaded.

Drying lamps are more commonly used in salons than at home; usually two are used together, one for the front and one for the back of your hair. Quartz driers are lightweight, hand-held driers that beam out infra-red rays to dry the hair. Salons often use hood driers; home versions of these are also available.

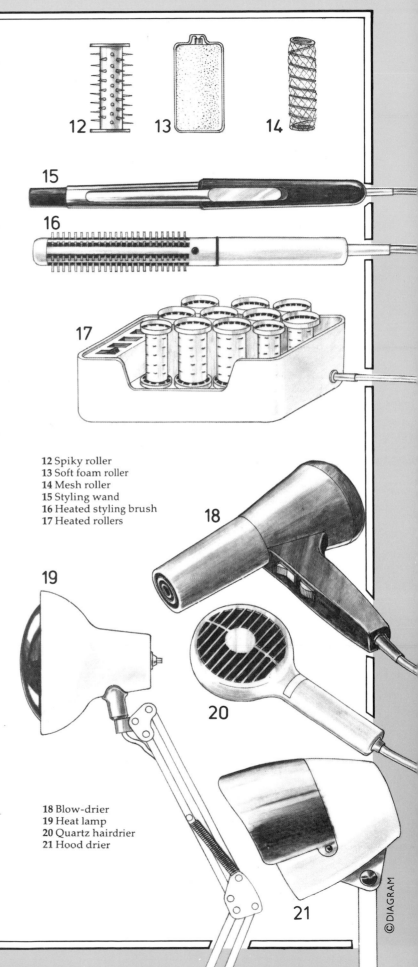

12 Spiky roller
13 Soft foam roller
14 Mesh roller
15 Styling wand
16 Heated styling brush
17 Heated rollers

18 Blow-drier
19 Heat lamp
20 Quartz hairdrier
21 Hood drier

Washing

Washing is one of the top priorities for keeping your hair looking at its best. Dirty or greasy hair looks lank and scruffy instead of shiny and full of movement. You can shampoo your hair every day if you wish but if you wash your hair this often you should use a very mild shampoo. Generally the rule is to wash your hair whenever it looks or feels dirty.

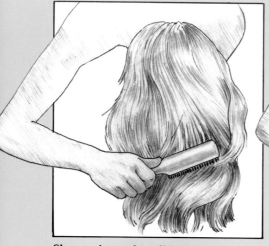

Shampooing and conditioning
1 Brush your hair through to get rid of any tangles and dirt from the scalp.

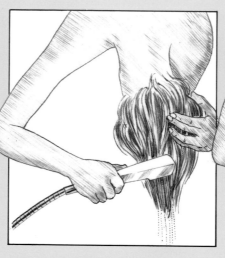

2 Wet the hair thoroughly, leaning over a bath or basin. Use a shower attachment to make sure the hair is wet all over.

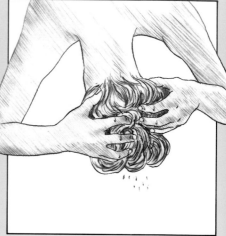

3 Pour a small amount of shampoo into your hand. Massage the hair well with your fingertips, starting at the scalp and working through to the ends.

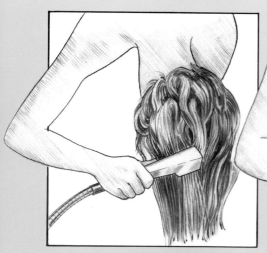

4 Rinse your hair thoroughly and check that there is no shampoo left in your hair.

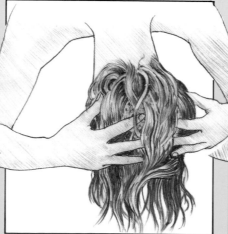

5 Squeeze out any excess moisture with your hands.

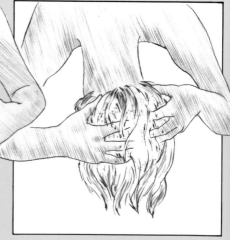

6 Rub a small amount of conditioner into the hair – not the scalp.

TYPES OF SHAMPOO

Shampoos are available in different forms to suit varying needs. You will probably need to experiment with different brands of shampoo to find just the right one for your hair.

Remember to look for a shampoo that suits your hair type; the label will say whether the shampoo is formulated for dry, greasy, flyaway, brittle, normal, or fine hair.

Hypoallergenic shampoos are for people with sensitive skin: they are unperfumed and are prepared with as few allergens (allergy-inducing substances) as possible.

Medicated shampoos are generally for hair that suffers from dandruff – the medication may not help the dandruff itself, but it will kill any bacteria that cling to the loose flakes of skin. True anti-dandruff shampoos contain an ingredient (usually zinc pyrithione) to dissolve away the flakes themselves. Anti-dandruff shampoos tend to be rather harsh, so don't use them every time you wash your hair – once a fortnight will probably keep your dandruff under control.

Frequent-wash shampoos are just what their name suggests – mild formulas for daily or very frequent hair-washing. Use only one application of shampoo if you wash your hair often, and you will avoid stripping away the hair's natural protection.

Single-application shampoos contain a water-softening ingredient so that you only need to wash and rinse the hair once. Some single-application shampoos need to be shaken vigorously before use to mix the ingredients thoroughly.

Conditioning shampoos attempt simultaneously to do the two very different tasks of washing and conditioning the hair with one product. You will probably find it better to use two separate products.

Organic shampoos are based on natural ingredients rather than chemicals.

Dry shampoos come in powder form and are based on talc or cornstarch. The powder is shaken onto the hair and gently rubbed in to distribute it; it absorbs excess grease and is then brushed out. Dry shampoos are not recommended for regular use, but they may be a boon in emergencies, or if you are ill in bed.

WASHING DIFFERENT HAIR TYPES

Oily hair should be washed frequently (every day if you wish) with one application of a mild shampoo and warm, rather than hot, water. A final rinse of clean water with a little vinegar or lemon juice will restore the acid/alkali balance of the hair.

Dry hair does not usually need to be washed as frequently as oily hair; use one application of a shampoo specially formulated for dry hair. Massage the scalp thoroughly and finish with a good conditioner (see pp. 152–153).

Normal hair simply needs to be washed with a balanced shampoo whenever it gets dirty.

Combination hair should be washed with a single application of a mild shampoo. Use a conditioner on just the ends of the hair.

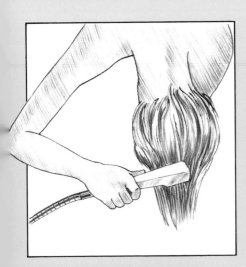

7 After a few minutes, rinse away the excess conditioner; don't be afraid to rinse thoroughly, as your hair will have absorbed all the conditioner it needs.

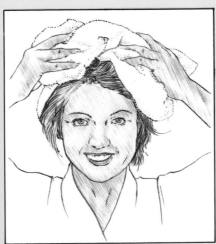

8 Blot the hair with a towel; never rub it, as the hair is at its weakest when wet.

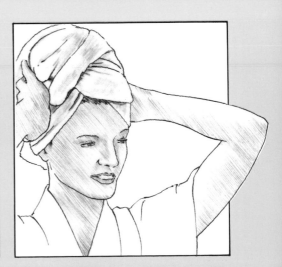

9 Wrap your hair in a towelling turban and leave it to absorb the moisture. When the hair is damp rather than wet, comb it through and dry in the usual way.

Conditioning and colouring

Very few of us are completely satisfied with our hair all of the time. Fortunately, these days we can choose from a wide range of safe, simple to use, and effective conditioners and colourants that can make all the difference.

CONDITIONING

The main purpose of any conditioner is to restore the electrical balance of the hair – many people find that if they don't use a conditioner their hair is charged with static electricity when it dries, which makes it difficult to control. Conditioners also smooth the scales of keratin so that the hair tangles less and dries with a better sheen. A conditioner, then, is a vital part of hair-care.
The most common conditioners are those for use with your shampoo: sometimes these are labelled "instant conditioners" or "creme rinse". Once the hair has been washed the conditioner is massaged in, left for a few minutes, and then rinsed off. A minute or two is all that the process takes, as by then the hairs have absorbed their fill: leaving the conditioner on for longer will not make any difference.
Other conditioners are deep-penetrating; these are useful for restoring your hair to good condition after too much holiday sun, or if your hair has been damaged by bleaching, tinting, perming, or over-drying. Some deep-penetrating conditioners, especially hot and cold oils, are applied before shampooing. Others are applied to clean, wet hair and left on for longer than routine conditioners, as they act in a different way.

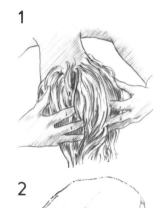
1

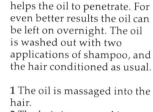
2

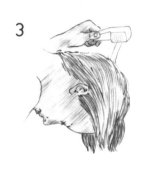
3

Hot oil conditioning
This can be done with special oils sold for the hair, or with other oils such as coconut or almond oil. The oil is warmed and then massaged into the hair. The oiled hair is wrapped in plastic, covered with a warm towel, and left for half an hour: the heat helps the oil to penetrate. For even better results the oil can be left on overnight. The oil is washed out with two applications of shampoo, and the hair conditioned as usual.

1 The oil is massaged into the hair.
2 The hair is wrapped in a warm towel.
3 The oil is washed out.

COLOURING

There are many ways of changing your hair colour, depending on its original shade and how long you want the effect to last.

Temporary rinses are the mildest form of hair colourant. They are applied to clean, wet hair, and the colour lasts until the next shampoo. Because they only coat each hair with colour, rather than altering the basic colour of the hair itself, they are most effective on light hair. They are useful for improving the look of permanently coloured hair between tinting sessions, or for helping to mask grey hair.

Semi-permanent colourants are left on clean, wet hair for 20–40 minutes before being rinsed out. The effects will last through 4–6 shampoos. Use these colourants to intensify your own hair colour or to lighten it by only one or two shades, e.g. to add auburn tones to dark hair, or a golden tone to mousy hair. Because these colourants contain complex chemicals, you should always do a test patch for allergies 24 hours before tinting your hair. And, of course, it is essential to read and follow the manufacturer's instructions to the letter.

Vegetable dyes are non-toxic and cannot harm your hair: in fact, many of them have a conditioning as well as a colouring effect. You must remember that they are less easy to control than modern chemical dyes – treat them with respect and change colour in easy stages, or you may regret the results, which are permanent! Henna has been used for centuries as a hair colourant, and can be obtained in many shades from golden brown to dark red. The henna powder (made from crushed henna leaves) is mixed to a paste and applied all over the hair. After 30–60 minutes it is rinsed out and the hair is washed. Always use rubber gloves when applying henna, or you will colour your hands as well as your hair. Henna is most effective on dark hair,

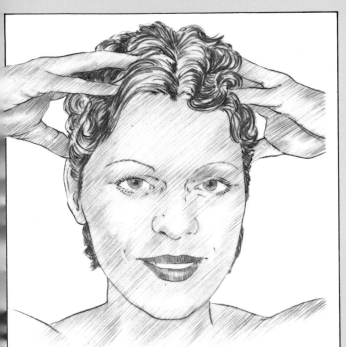

SCALP MASSAGE

Scalp massage is a wonderfully relaxing treatment, which loosens a taut scalp, improves circulation, and stimulates healthy new hair growth. Massage your head before you wash your hair, perhaps using a little aromatic oil to scent and condition the hair at the same time.

Use the pads of the fingertips, not the nails, and make small circular movements all over your head with the fingers and thumbs of both hands. Move the scalp as you massage, rather than moving the fingers. Cover every inch of the scalp, but pay special attention to any areas that are tense, such as the base of the neck. A circular rubber massage brush can be used for scalp massage instead of the fingers.

while infusions of camomile or marigold work best on fair hair, lightening and warming the natural colour.

Permanent tints actually alter the structure of the hair, so having one should be regarded as a serious step, and should only be taken if you are prepared to spend time and money having the roots touched up. These are the colourants to use if you want to make any major changes in your hair colour. For the best results, have permanent tinting done in a salon by a professional colourist. If you do decide to do it yourself at home, follow the manufacturer's instructions very carefully, test patch for allergies, and test the tint on a few strands cut from your own hair to see what the finished colour will be. Remember that permanently tinted hair can be very susceptible to damage, and treat it carefully.

LIGHTENING AND HIGHLIGHTING

If you want to permanently change your hair colour to a total blonde, it will need to be bleached (to remove your natural colour) and then retinted (to give the finished colour). This is drastic treatment, and the repeated applications needed to retouch the roots can cause terrible damage to your hair. Most reputable hairdressers will suggest gentler alternative ways of producing a blonde effect, by streaking, highlighting, or tipping the hair. These techniques do not use bleach, but a chemical lightener that is much kinder to the hair. The effect can be very natural, and because there is no hard line at the roots, retouching is only needed every 4–6 months. Highlighting, streaking, and tipping need not be confined to blonde effects. They can be used to introduce other colours into your hair – red streaks in dark hair, perhaps, or even pink, green, or other "crazy" colours. And you can also have lowlights, where a colour darker than your natural shade is streaked into your hair. Whichever you choose, have it done professionally at a salon unless you are very skilled at home colouring.

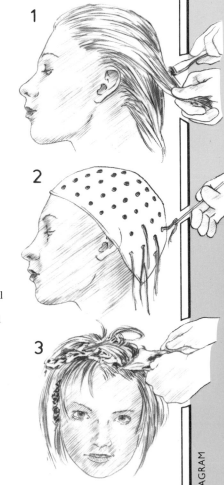

Streaking and tipping
Streaking involves painting on lines of lightener (**1**), usually in places where the hair would be naturally bleached by the sun. The longer the lightener is left in place before rinsing off, the lighter the final tone of the hair. Tipping is a similar technique to streaking, but the lightener is applied only to the very ends of the hair: this can look particularly good on short, feathery cuts.

Highlighting
Two different techniques are used to separate off the thin sections of hair to be highlighted. You may be asked to put on a plastic cap, and small sections of hair will be drawn through holes in the cap (**2**). The lightener will then be applied to these sections, left to act, and then rinsed off. Alternatively, a strand of hair may be lifted onto a piece of tinfoil and then painted with lightener (**3**). The hair is left wrapped in the foil until the lightener has taken effect, when it is rinsed out.

©DIAGRAM

153

Cutting

The cut of your hair should show it off to the best advantage whatever its characteristics. A good hairdresser will be able to find many different styles that will show it off to good effect. Hair should always be cut wet; it may then be re-trimmed dry to correct any minor faults or irregularities. A cut usually lasts for about six weeks in good shape before it begins to lose its definition as the individual hairs grow at different speeds. Whatever the specific style chosen, your hair will probably be cut in one of two basic styles: blunt cut or layered cut.

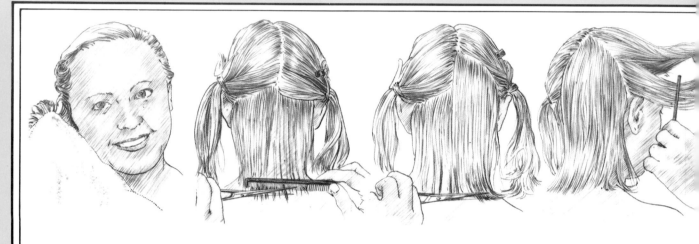

Basic blunt cut
1 The hair is washed, conditioned and combed through.

2 Most of the hair is clipped back out of the way from a centre parting, and the lowest level at the back is combed down and cut straight.

3 The next section is brought down and cut level with the first.

4 Some of the side hair is brought down and cut level with the hair at the back.

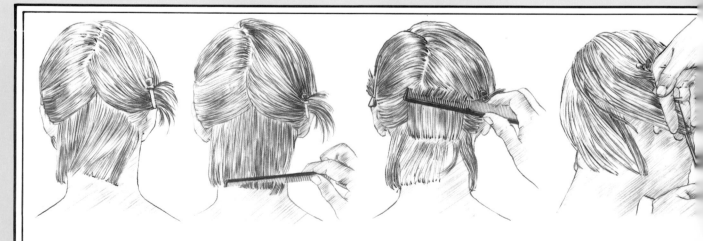

Basic layer cut
1 After the hair has been washed, towelled dry and combed, a centre parting is made and most of the hair clipped back out of the way.

2 The hair is combed down to the nape of the neck and cut, using a comb to hold it in position.

3 After the baseline has been established, some more hair is combed to the back and cut in an arched shape.

4 The lower side sections are brought forward and cut to form the side edges of the style.

BLUNT CUTS

Blunt cuts style the hair so that it is all the same length at any particular point of the hairstyle. The cut may be a short bob, a shoulder-length fall of hair, or even a waist-length style, and the hair may be cut with or without bangs. Whatever the style, the ends of the hair will all be cut to the same level. Blunt cuts look their best on straight hair, as the style stays in place more easily, but women with wavy hair can often have their hair cut and blow-dried into an even cut such as a shoulder-length bob or a pageboy cut.

LAYER CUTS

There are many, many variations of the layer cut, but the basic technique is the same. The hair is cut shorter at the top and sides, and left longer at the back, or it may be cut very short around the back and sides to give a boyish look. Gel and mousse can be used to make the hair spiky or full; it can be "scrunch-dried" to give a random effect, or it can be blow-dried or tonged into curls, waves, or a sleek head of hair. Layered cuts of different sorts can be done on any kind of hair.

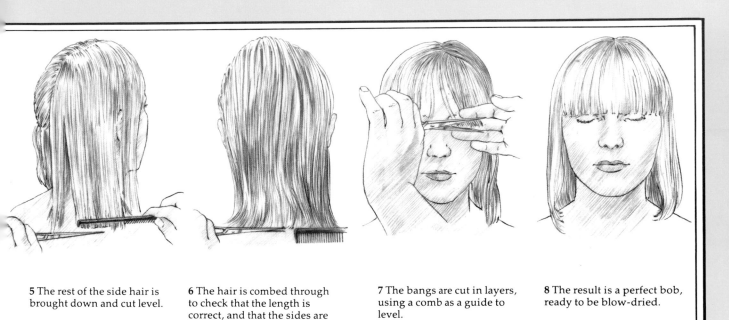

5 The rest of the side hair is brought down and cut level.

6 The hair is combed through to check that the length is correct, and that the sides are cut level.

7 The bangs are cut in layers, using a comb as a guide to level.

8 The result is a perfect bob, ready to be blow-dried.

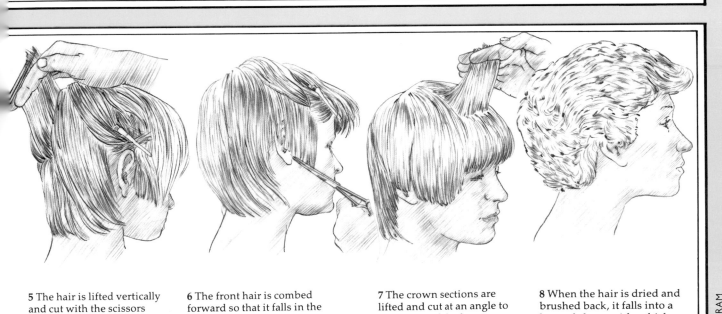

5 The hair is lifted vertically and cut with the scissors angled toward the crown of the head.

6 The front hair is combed forward so that it falls in the natural growth line, then cut in a curve from the cheek to the ear.

7 The crown sections are lifted and cut at an angle to achieve a soft look.

8 When the hair is dried and brushed back, it falls into a layered shape with a thick, natural look.

Setting and perming 1

Setting and perming can both be used to add extra body, bounce, or curl to your hair. Setting is a temporary measure – the effects can last for anything from a few hours or until you next wash your hair, depending on your hair type and the setting technique you use. Perming, as the name suggests, is permanent – the effects last as long as the permed hair lasts.

ROLLER SETTING
Rollers have more holding power than heated setting appliances. Hair that is naturally curly or wavy will curl more tightly, and needs larger rollers than fine or straight hair. Only a small section of hair should be wound onto each roller, or your hair will take a very long time to dry and the finished effect will be uneven.

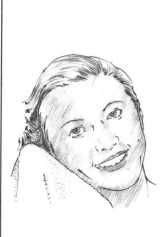 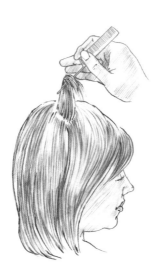 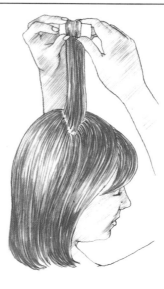 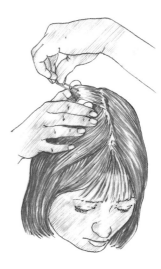

Standard set for body and bounce
1 Wash your hair and towel it dry, leaving it slightly damp. A setting lotion or gel applied at this stage will help keep the set in place.

2 Use the tail of a rattail comb to divide off a small, rectangular section of hair, and comb it through.

3 Hold the hair out from the head, straight but not stretched, and wind the ends round a medium-sized roller.

4 Wind the strand evenly and firmly round the roller, down to the scalp. Secure with a hairpin pushed in at 45° to the scalp. If the hair is rolled under, the pin points up, and vice versa.

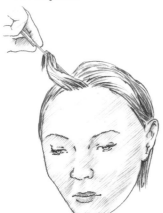 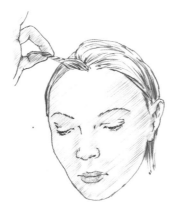 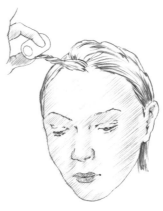 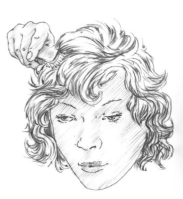

Set for tight curls
1 Take a section of your hair as you would for a normal set.

2 Twist the section of hair in a clockwise direction with your fingers.

3 Wind the twisted section of hair round the roller in the usual way, and secure.

4 When the hair is brushed out it will be tightly curled; the tighter the twist, the tighter the curl.

SETTING AGENTS

The styles of today are easier than ever to keep in shape. Natural looks are the order of the day – no longer do hairdressers set the hair into regimented rows of cylindrical curls. Sets are used instead to give the hair life, thickness, wave or soft curl.

Setting lotion is a thin liquid that is often used in roller setting. It is combed through the hair before the rollers are put in, and holds the curls in place once the hair is dry.

Setting mousses have created quite a revolution in hair styling in recent years; they give short styles shape and body. The mousse is sprayed onto the hand from an aerosol, spread through the hair, and then the hair is blow-dried into shape.

Gels can be used to sleek back the hair for a very streamlined look, or to hold shape in spiky styles. They are also good for holding down wisps of wavy hair if you want a smooth finish.

Hairsprays these days are fine, light, and virtually invisible, and very easy to brush out. They can be very useful for holding a style in place, especially outdoors.

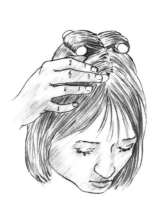

5 Insert rollers in the same way all around the top of the hair.

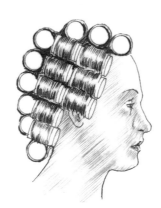

6 Set the rest of the hair in even sections, working from one side round the back to the other side.

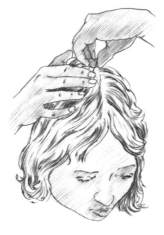

7 Dry the hair with a blow-drier, or leave to dry naturally. When fully dry, remove the pins and rollers.

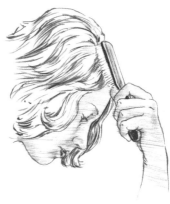

8 Brush through gently to leave a full, soft curl.

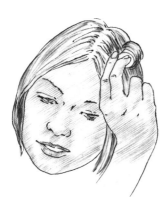

Extra body for soft hair
Putting in rollers in different directions gives extra body.
1 Divide the hair down the middle and roll sections of the top hair upward toward the crown of the head.

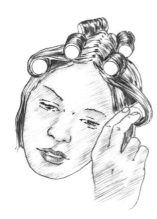

2 Roll the next layer of rollers downward.

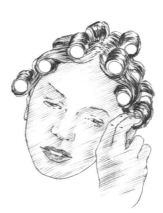

3 Roll the bottom layer of rollers upward.

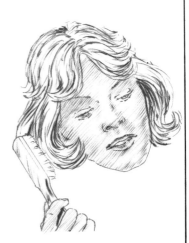

4 When brushed out, the alternate directions of curl will give the hair extra body and movement.

SETTING WITHOUT ROLLERS

If you prefer not to use rollers, there are several alternative ways of setting your hair while it is damp.

Ragrolling is a traditional but still effective hair-curling method that is particularly good for producing ringlets in long hair when there is too much to wind around rollers. Long strands of hair are twisted tightly and then bound with strips of cotton rag to keep the twist in until the hair is dry.

Foam rods can be used on long or short hair; the hair is twirled around the foam, then the foam rod is bent back on itself to secure it during the drying process.

Pincurling is used for producing random curls on short hair, or ringlets on longer hair. A strand of hair is twisted very tightly until it loops back on itself, and this knot of hair is secured with a metal clip during drying.

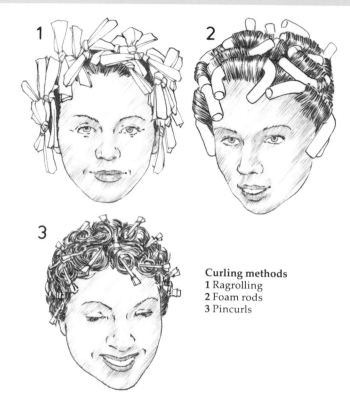

Curling methods
1 Ragrolling
2 Foam rods
3 Pincurls

PERMING

If you know that you want more than an occasional wave or set in your hair, you may consider a permanent wave. This is a serious step, as the hair is restructured to a completely new shape with chemicals and setting rods; the effect is irreversible. Perms can be done at home, but it is much safer to have the process done at a salon – your hair is too important to take risks with. Your hairdresser will be able to advise you on the best kind of perm to suit your hair's length, texture, and condition, and will make sure that all the perming rods are positioned properly. The shape of the rods, the condition of the hair, and the

length of time that the rods are left in position all contribute to the final effect of the perm. Different types of perm are used to achieve different effects.

Ordinary perms are designed to give an even, all-over curl to short or long hair.

Body perms or demi-waves are soft perms shaped on large rods that produce waves rather than tight curls.

Partial perming can be done if you just want one section of your hair curly – perhaps bubbly curls on the crown with short straight hair at the back and sides. Partial perming can also be used to even out your hair if part of your hair is naturally

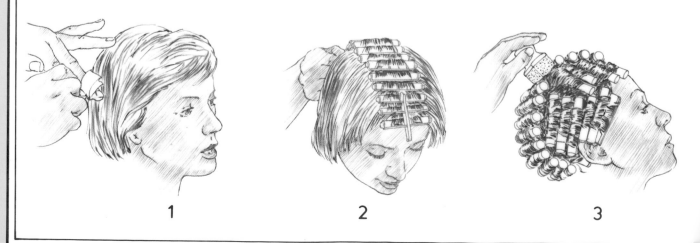

1   2   3

DRY SETTING

Your hair can be restyled while it is dry to provide variety in between washes, or the style can be brushed in during the drying process. Heated rollers, styling wands, and heated brushes are all methods of quickly putting curl into dry hair; the hair is wrapped around the appliance for a short time so that the heat sets the curl. These methods can be used for anything from smoothing out a pageboy bob to creating a pile of curls on the top of the head.

Blow-drying is a skill all to itself, generally used to give shape and body rather than tight curl. Some blow-driers are equipped with brush and comb attachments so that the hair is brushed into shape and dried in the same action. Others are used to direct heat onto a section of hair that is being held in place with a brush or comb. The hair can be flicked up, turned under, waved, or loosely curled with the blow-drying method.

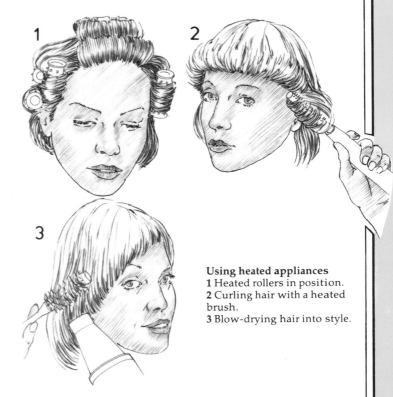

Using heated appliances
1 Heated rollers in position.
2 Curling hair with a heated brush.
3 Blow-drying hair into style.

curly and other parts naturally straight.

Relaxing or straightening is perming in reverse; frizzy or wavy hair is kept straight during the perming process. Straightening is a fiercer process than ordinary perming, and tends to have a more detrimental effect on the hair's condition.

Root perms are used to provide body to your hair near the roots. The ends of the hair are protected, and only the parts near the scalp are permed.

CARING FOR PERMED HAIR

Perming should only be done on healthy hair that is in good condition and newly cut. Ask your hairdresser's advice about perming if your hair has been coloured or still has some of a previous perm left in it.

After your perm your hair is more vulnerable — try not to use a hairdrier for several days after the perm to give it time to settle. Greasy hair may well improve in looks, with more bounce and less lankness, but normal hair will be drier and more prone to splitting; make sure that it is always well conditioned.

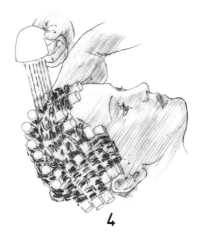

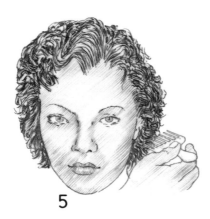

Steps in perming
1 Each piece of hair is carefully sectioned off, and the ends are wrapped in tissue.
2 The strands of hair are rolled around the perming rods.
3 The hair is softened with a waving solution, to make it more receptive to a change in shape.
4 The waving solution is rinsed off. A neutralising solution is applied that makes the hair firm again so that it takes on its new shape.
5 The rods are removed and the hair brushed into shape.

Drying

Unless you have a "wash and wear" style (when you can just leave your hair to dry naturally), how you dry your hair will play an important part in creating your finished hairstyle.

DRYING TECHNIQUES

Methods of drying vary with the final effect desired, with the cut and length of the hair, and with the setting technique used.

Hand-held or hood driers are used to dry hair that has been set in rollers, pincurls, etc. These sets can be left to dry naturally but heat makes the process much quicker and also helps to strengthen the curl in the hair. Salons may use heat lamps or quartz driers instead of more conventional driers.

Finger-drying may be used for short, ragged, curly, or spiky cuts. The hair is simply pushed into place with the fingers and dried with a hand-held drier.

Scrunch drying is used for random curl and wave: a handful of hair is held tightly scrunched in the hand while the heat is directed onto the hair between the fingers.

Blow drying is used to introduce curl and body into the hair: this could be to smooth under a bob, flick bangs to the side, give a gentle wave to long hair, or shape the whole of a short hairstyle. Use a full- or half-radial styling brush to shape your hair as you dry it with a hand-held drier, or choose one of the special driers with brush or comb attachments that shape and dry the hair at the same time.

BASIC BLOW-DRYING TECHNIQUE

Before you begin blow-drying, wrap your hair in a towel for 10 minutes to absorb most of the moisture. Hair does not begin to take on a shape until it is nearly dry, so blow-drying wet hair is just wasted effort.

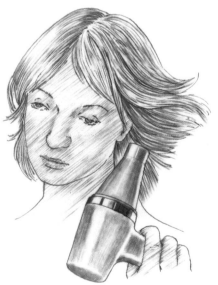

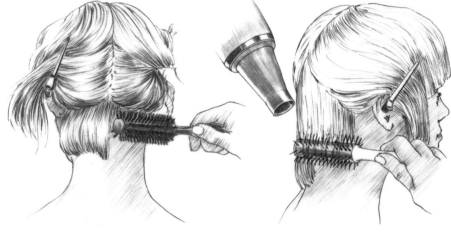

1 Roughly blow-dry the hair all over the head until it is just very slightly damp. Some special blow-dry conditioners can be added at this stage.

2 Use metal clips to hold back hair that is not to be worked on yet. Beginning with the centre back, roll up the hair in 5cm sections and direct the heat toward the roots, moving it steadily across the rolled up hair. Lift the brush to give more bounce and to speed up the drying process.

3 Unpin other sections and gradually blend in the layers as you dry. Allow the quills of the brush to grip the hair at the ends and turn under with a steady roll of the wrist.

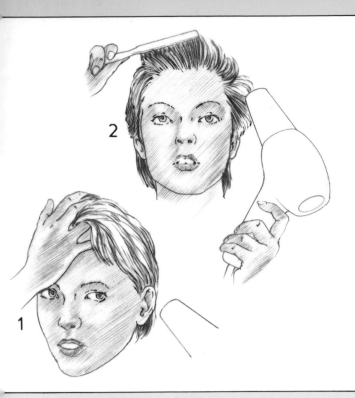

TIPS FOR BLOW-DRYING

Always work with small sections of hair; they are easier to control. Keep hair you are not working on out of the way by clipping it back with hairpins.

For sleek, straight hair, brush downward from the crown in long strokes.

To straighten frizzy hair, catch the ends tightly in a brush and hold the hair out from the head; direct the heat from the top.

For a full, straight effect, brush your hair forward from the nape of the neck, put your head down, and blow-dry the hair upside down.

For a fairly tight curl, wind your hair in sections round a fine brush and direct the heat onto it as if it were on a roller.

To give layered hair a feathery effect, direct the hot air across the hair from the side.

1 Styling the hair with a drier and fingers.

2 Styling the hair with a drier and a styling brush.

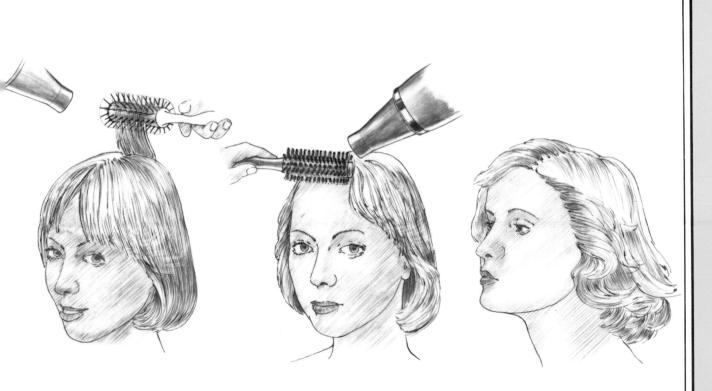

4 Give the top hair extra lift by rolling it up closer to the roots, but always leave about 2·5 cm unrolled so that the hair is not damaged.

5 Brush the side hair away from the parting, turning the hair gently under while you direct the heat at the top. Brush the bangs into shape and dry.

6 The finished style should have a smooth appearance, with no rolls of hair that have not been incorporated into the finished style. Leave the hair to cool completely before you give it a final brush, or you will brush out the curl.

Hair problems and treatments

Few people have hair that is always in good condition and full of bounce and body. Almost everyone has to cope at some time with hair that is greasy, lank, dry, damaged or out of condition, or with split ends or dandruff. Your hair is on show all the time, so you want it to look at its best – any problems should be dealt with as soon as they occur.

DRY HAIR

Dry hair is vulnerable and easily damaged because it lacks the normal protective coat of sebum. Sebum smooths the keratin scales on the surface of the hair so that the hair is glossy and in good condition – lack of sebum means the hair's surface is rough, and the hair easily becomes tangled, knotted, and split. If dry hair is your problem, always use a shampoo and rich conditioner specially formulated for dry hair, and use fingertip scalp massage during washing to stimulate the sebaceous glands.

OILY HAIR

Oily hair looks lank and lifeless, and picks up dust and dirt very easily. Frequent washing with a mild shampoo is necessary, but use warm rather than hot water so that the sebaceous glands are not overstimulated.

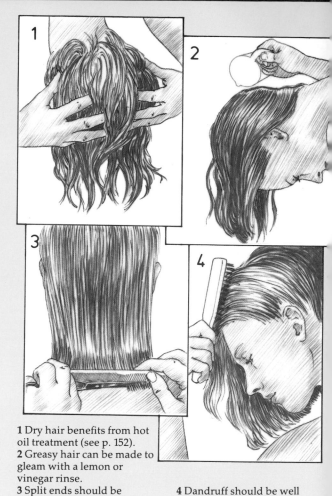

1 Dry hair benefits from hot oil treatment (see p. 152).
2 Greasy hair can be made to gleam with a lemon or vinegar rinse.
3 Split ends should be trimmed off regularly.
4 Dandruff should be well brushed out.

HAIR LOSS

The average person may lose around 100 hairs a day and not notice the difference, but for some people hair loss can become a problem. Hair loss may occur as a result of the aging process (although balding is only rarely a problem for women), or as the result of disease or some other physiological factor. Prolonged illness may cause a deterioration in the general state of the hair, possibly including extra hair loss. Some forms of medical treatment (e.g. chemotherapy) can also cause the hair to fall out. In all these cases you should seek expert professional advice. Between them, your doctor and your hairdresser should be able to advise you on what treatments you may need, what regrowth of hair you can expect, and the best way to deal with the problem in the meantime – perhaps by wearing additional hair or a wig.

Careless treatment can also cause hair loss. If the hair is constantly pulled tight into the same style, the hair roots may weaken and the hair may fall out: the condition is called traction alopecia. Overprocessing – perhaps too harsh or too frequent perming or relaxing – can make the hair so brittle that it breaks off at or near the scalp. Little can be done to restore the hair's condition in this case: if it happens to you, have your hair cut short and wait for new, healthy hair to grow.

FRAGILE HAIR

This is usually the result of too much perming, tinting, and colouring, or too frequent use of heated rollers, driers and tongs. The protective surface of the hair becomes damaged, making the hair very vulnerable. It needs very gentle treatment to restore it to health. Use a wide-tooth comb that does not tug or tear your hair, and wear you hair in a simple style that does not need a lot of handling. Use a rich conditioning pack on the hair twice a week, and avoid blow-driers and heated rollers. It will usually take about three months to get the hair back into condition.

SPLIT ENDS

Fragile hair splits easily, but split ends can also occur in hair – especially long hair – that is in otherwise good condition. They are usually the result of not treating your hair with enough care – using spiky rollers carelessly, perhaps, or using heated hair appliances too frequently. If your hair tends to split, use a brush with well spaced rounded nylon quills in preference to a bristle brush, and make sure that you use a protective conditioner before blow-drying your hair. Most important of all, have your hair trimmed regularly to remove the split ends, as this will prevent the split travelling up the hair.

DANDRUFF

In mild cases of dandruff, small flakes of skin appear in the hair. This may be the result of using harsh hair products, or an accompaniment to general dry skin and dry hair. Vigorous brushing with a gentle bristle brush will stimulate the scalp and remove the dandruff; scalp massage will help bring more nutrients to the scalp to feed the skin and hair. In more severe cases of dandruff, the flakes of skin are coated with sebum and may be infected: special medicated and anti-dandruff shampoos should be included in your hair-washing regime to deal with the problem.

COLOUR LOSS

Grey hair occurs as the body ages: the hair follicles gradually stop producing pigment in the hair shaft so that it emerges colourless. Nothing can be done to halt the process. Some people are quite happy with grey hair as it appears, others prefer to disguise it, and still others choose to enhance it with streaks or highlights. A colour tint or rinse is the best way of disguising greying hair, giving a gentle overall colouring that doesn't look artificial. Choose your shade carefully: as you get older your face loses colour, so even if you had black hair before you went grey, it could look strange on you now. Grey hair can sometimes become yellowy, which looks unattractive, but this can be corrected with an ash rinse. Special conditioners are now formulated for grey hair, and they include a mild colour rinse to improve the hair's appearance.

SCALP PROBLEMS

There are a number of skin conditions that can affect the scalp as well as the skin on the rest of the body. They require professional medical treatment, and you should consult your doctor if you suspect that you suffer from either dermatitis, eczema, psoriasis, or a fungal infection (all described on p. 78).
A less serious but equally unpleasant scalp problem can be caused by lice. These small parasites love clean hair and lay their eggs there. The first sign of their presence is usually an itching scalp, and on closer inspection the eggs or nits are visible. Treatment involves applying a special lotion to kill the lice and using a "nit comb" to remove the eggs from the hair.

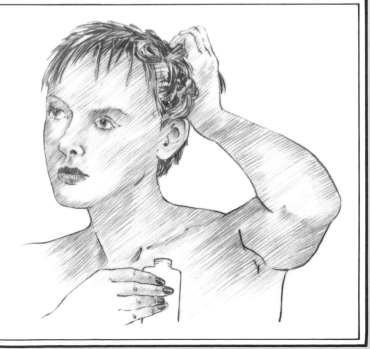

©DIAGRAM

Wigs and hairpieces

If you want to change the appearance of your hair temporarily, perhaps to try out a new hairstyle, a different hair colour, or simply because your hair looks a mess after a day at the beach, then a wig could be the answer. Nowadays most wigs and hairpieces are made of very realistic man-made fibres. It is still possible to have wigs made from real hair, but they are very expensive and need professional care.

CHOOSING A WIG

If you want your wig to look really natural, go to a specialist wig supplier where they can offer you both professional advice and a wide choice of styles and qualities. A good quality wig is made with more hair in it than is really necessary: this means that it can be thinned and trimmed to suit you perfectly. Choose your style of wig very carefully, as styles that look good on your own hair may not be as suitable in a wig, and may simply emphasise the fact that it is artificial.

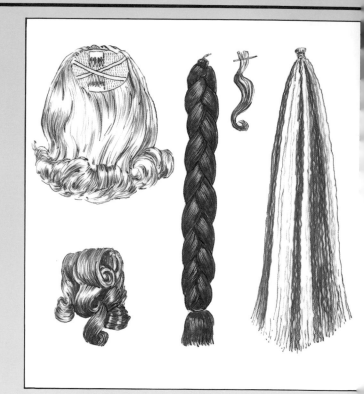

PUTTING ON A WIG

When you wear a wig, it is worth spending time putting it on properly. Your hair should be well flattened, or the wig will appear bumpy and uneven. One common mistake among wig-wearers is to put the wig too far forward, giving a very strange hairline. If the wig has bangs, these can be used to soften any harsh line on the forehead; if not, put the wig back a little from your natural hairline and blend in a few of your own hairs to soften the effect.

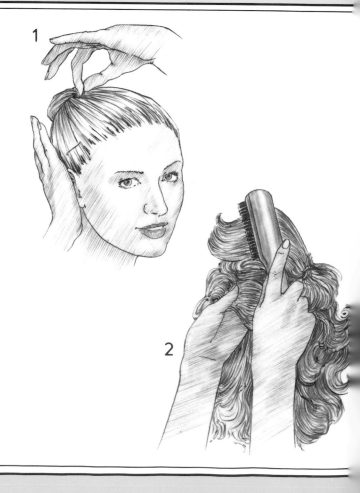

1. Flatten your own hair thoroughly so that the wig will lie well. Loop long hair back in loose, flat pincurls, and comb short hair back and hold it with a row of hairpins across the crown.

2 Hold the wig in front of you upside down and give it a thorough brushing to remove any tangles.

3 Pull the wig on from the front, making sure the centre of the wig is in the centre of your forehead.

4 Check that none of your own hair has escaped round the back and sides. Tease through some hair at the front if you want to soften the hairline. Secure the wig with hairgrips, as inconspicuously as possible.

5 Arrange your hair in the desired style, and brush very lightly so that the wig is not dislodged.

TYPES OF FALSE HAIR

Strictly a wig is a full head of hair that fits right over the scalp and hides your own hair completely: the hairs are stitched onto a mesh base that is pulled over your own hair like a cap. Other effects can be achieved with partial hairpieces in the shape of falls, topknots, fine or thick braids, etc. Some people like to keep their options open when they have their hair cut from long to short, and to have the cut pieces of their own hair made into a long fall or formed into braids for augmenting a shorter style. Of course all kinds of wigs and hairpieces are useful for people whose hair has been damaged through chemical treatments, such as chemotherapy, or through conditions such as alopecia. Some people's hair is very fine, especially at the back: in this case the styles can be augmented by carefully positioned hair falls, chosen to blend in with the natural hair. Very frizzy afro hair may not grow very long, and in this case too a fall of hair provides some options for a longer style. Thick and thin braids can be used for all kinds of exotic styles suitable for special occasions, or simply for taking a lot of the trouble out of styles requiring time-consuming braiding.

WIG AND HAIR CARE

Synthetic wigs need only the minimum of care, but they should be protected from dust and washed regularly. All wigs will keep their shape best if they are stored on a wig stand, and they should be kept well away from sources of heat. A full wig keeps in body heat, allowing it to build up on the scalp. If you wear a wig regularly, you will find that this heat makes your own hair become very lank. Wash your hair and scalp every day, and wash your wig every few days in warm water.

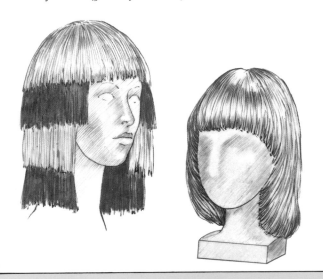

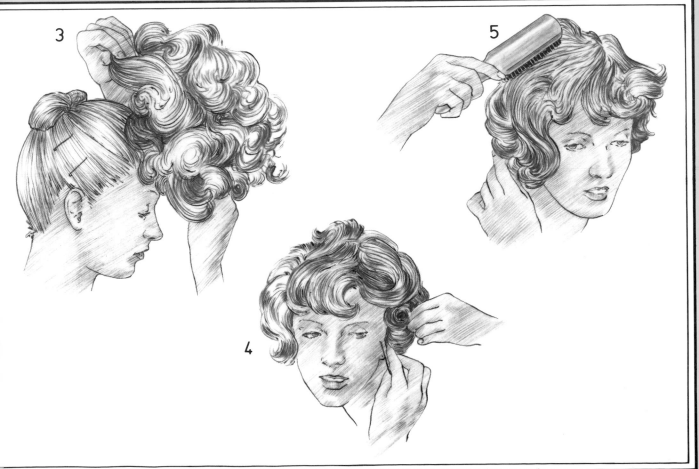

©DIAGRAM

Choosing a hairstyle 1

The hair style you choose can make or mar your looks. It may flatter your face or draw attention to poorer features, emphasise your character or be out of keeping with your attitudes and lifestyles. It's worth giving your hairstyle some careful thought: even the most marvellous hair needs to be cut and styled carefully.

PRIORITIES

You will need to sort out your own personal priorities for choosing one hairstyle above another. For example, does your lifestyle make special demands of your hairstyle? If you are a busy career woman always in the public eye, you may need a style that can be maintained easily and that always looks good with the minimum of care. Or you may need an adaptable style that can be swiftly altered from an efficient, businesslike look to something glamorous or extra-special. Manageability is an important consideration. If you swim or play sport regularly, you need an easy-care "wash and wear" style, so that you don't need to spend hours every day with a brush and hairdrier. If you lead a busy life you won't have much spare time to spend on styling your hair. But if time is no problem you may be able to opt for a more elaborate style for everyday wear. Economic factors are important. It is expensive to go to a salon every few weeks to have an

elaborate style reshaped, so you may want a simpler cut that you can trim yourself. Of course your own preference for long, short, or medium-length hair will also come into the reckoning. In some occupations, the hair must be swept back neatly all the time – your style will have to be chosen with this in mind. It also needs to suit your personality: a bubbly crimp falling seductively over one eye may look fantastic on a sultry model, but could be too much on a shy office worker. Your stature is another consideration. If you are plump, tall, and big-boned, a short, close-cropped style will make your head look very small in proportion to the rest of your body. Conversely, if you are tiny and fine-boned, a thick mass of curls could make you look top-heavy.

FACE SHAPE

The shape of your face (see pp. 106–107) is bound to influence the hairstyle you choose. Your aim will generally be to play down some features and emphasise others so that your face shape looks balanced. For example, if your face is too wide at the forehead, cheekbones, or jaw, your hairstyle should play down those areas rather than emphasising them.

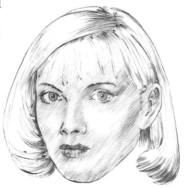 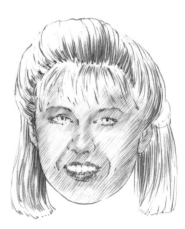

Square face
If your face is square or rectangular, you should be looking for a style that detracts from the angles. Wispy bangs, gentle side partings, curls, and waves around the ears will soften the lines. Your jaw will probably be quite broad, so avoid blunt cuts that finish on your jawline.

Round face
Styles swept back from your face, or lots of full curls all over your head, will simply emphasise your face's round shape. Give more height with fullness at the crown and shorter sides, or give more length with shoulder-length curls or bobs.

HAIR CHARACTERISTICS

Although hairdressers can do a great deal to overcome some of your hair's characteristics, there will always be some styles that are easier to do on your type of hair than others.

Your quantity of hair is one consideration – do you have a thick head of hair, or is there really very little of it? Thick hair can be "thinned" by careful cutting to reduce its body, or the thickness can be used to full effect for luxuriant curls or chunky short cuts. If your hair is not very thick it can be given the appearance of more body by layered cuts, the careful use of mousses and blow-drying, or by root or full perming.

Your hair's texture is another consideration. Is your hair coarse or fine, or somewhere in the middle? If it is coarse, conditioners may help to smooth it down and make it more manageable. Hair sprays will help hold your style in place, but your hair may simply not be adaptable enough for some styles. Fine hair can be given extra body by some of the chemicals used in hair colourants – because these actually lift the keratin scales on the hair they fatten each hair out a little, and so give more body overall. Fine hair often tends to be very straight as well, but a demi-wave can give it more lift and body, as can setting lotions, gels, and mousses.

Your hair's formation as it grows is something that cannot be changed, because it depends on the shape of your hair follicle. Of course the hair shafts themselves can be altered by perming, straightening, etc, but the new hair will still grow out in the old shape. If your hair is very straight and smooth you may want to play on that and choose a style that relies on the perfect lie of every hair – or you may want to alter its shape with a set or perm to introduce movement. If your hair is wavy or curly, again you can emphasise this feature or play it down. Blow-drying and setting can be used to make sure it waves just the way you want it to rather than at random. Frizzy hair is perhaps the least adaptable of all: it is best to choose a cut that uses the crinkly shape rather than trying to eradicate it.

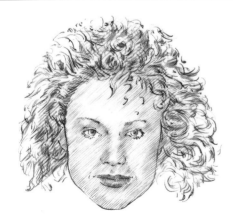

Long face
If your face is long, a style that adds width will suit you best. This could include thick, straight-cut bangs, curls or waves at the side, or layered cuts to add fullness. Avoid long, straight hair, or any styles that add height to the crown.

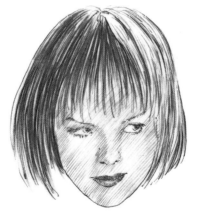

Oval face
This is the perfect face shape for any style. Keep your hairstyle simple so that it doesn't detract from the good balance of your features.

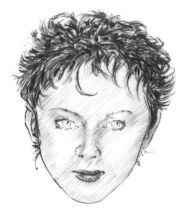

Diamond-shaped face
Width at the cheekbones is the problem with a diamond-shaped face, so avoid any style that gives fullness here. Sleek styles ending in shoulder-length waves or short cuts with fullness on the crown will be the most flattering.

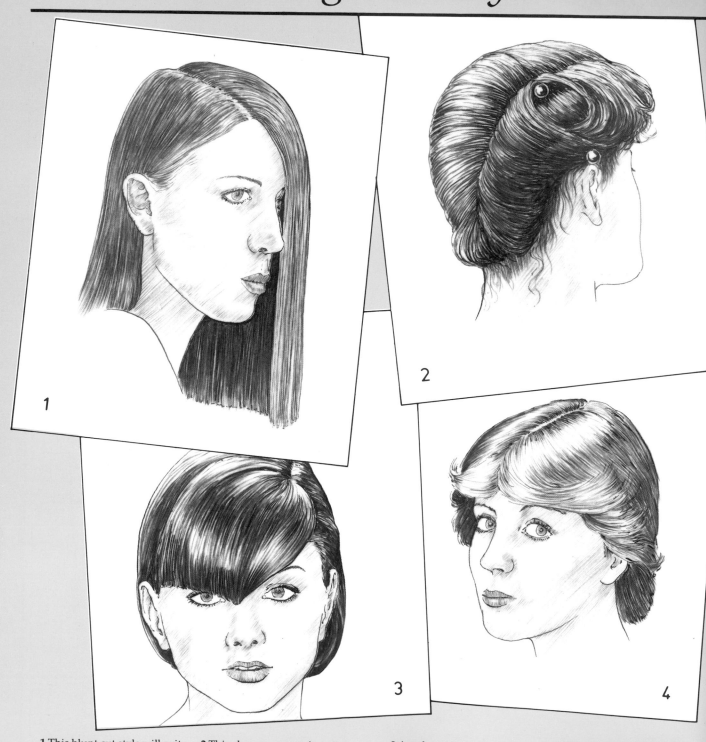

1 This blunt cut style will suit you if you have a round or an oval face, and fine, straight hair of medium thickness. The length means that the cut is versatile enough to be worn in different styles for different occasions. It will need regular cutting to keep it in perfect condition and to remove any split ends.

2 This shows one way in which style **1** can be adapted for a formal occasion – a variation on the classic French pleat. Fine hair can be difficult to keep in place when you put it up: give it some help with setting mousse, gel, or hairspray.

3 Another style for fine, straight hair of medium thickness, but this time for a diamond shape face. Geometric cuts like this one need precision cutting on hair that is in superb condition.

4 The same type of hair again, but this time in a layer cut that is suitable for either a long or an oval face. This is an easy care, easy to wear style. The flicked sides can easily be blow-dried into place, or shaped on dry hair with heated tongs or rollers.

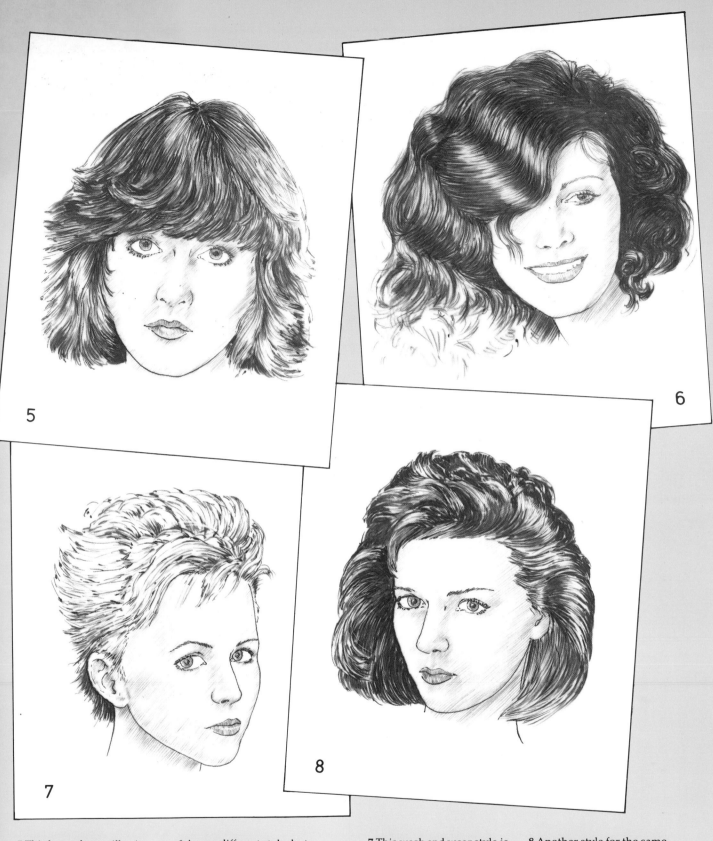

5

6

7

8

5 This layered cut will suit you if you have an oval or a long face, and "medium" hair – of medium thickness and neither too fine nor too coarse. Hair with a slight natural wave can be cut directly into this style, but if you have totally straight hair it will need a light perm first.

6 A very different style, but suitable for the same type of hair and face shape as style **5**. The deep wave over the eye could be pinned back for work, and then released for a more glamorous evening style.

7 This wash and wear style is for you if you have a round or diamond shape face, and fairly thick, fairly coarse hair with a slight wave. It would also be suitable on medium hair that has been body permed. Setting gel could be used to give extra height or for a spiky effect.

8 Another style for the same type of hair as in style **7**, but this time for a square face. This style could be blow dried into place, or set on rollers. The hair is long enough to allow the style to be easily changed for different occasions.

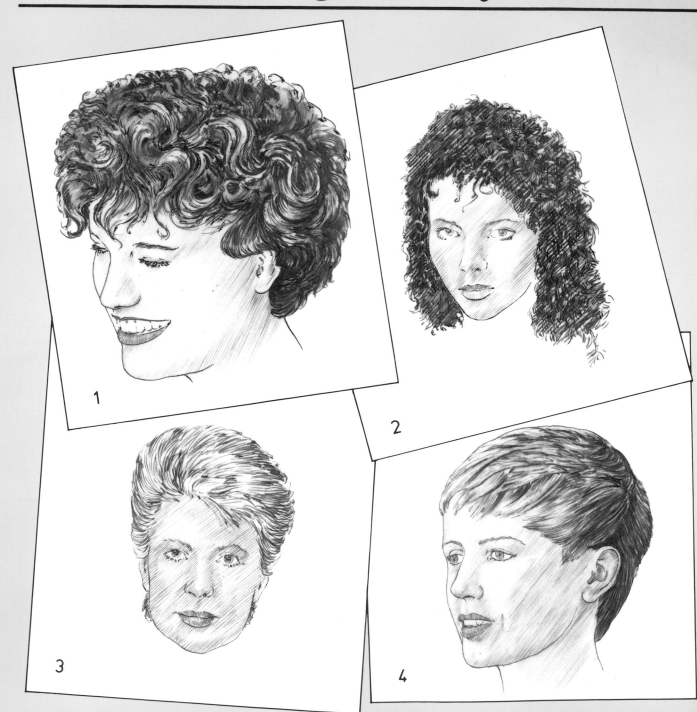

1 This style is for you if you have a round or an oval face, and really thick, coarse hair. Your hair should have plenty of natural curl, or you will need a very curly perm. Once permed, this will be a very easy style to look after – simply wash, condition, and leave to dry. Use a wide-toothed Afro comb to lift the curls.

2 Similar hair to style **1**, but in a style suitable for nearly all face shapes except a long face. To look good in this style, your hair must be shiny and in superb condition: use a spray-on conditioner on your hair when it is dry as well as your normal after-shampoo conditioner.

3 This style looks particularly good if your hair has been highlighted or if you are beginning to go grey. It is suitable for coarse, thick hair with some natural wave, and for a square, oval, or round face.

4 If you have baby fine, thin, straight hair, an oval or diamond shape face, and a small, neat head, try this feathery, layer cut style. It would look particularly good with the ends of the hair tipped with colour.

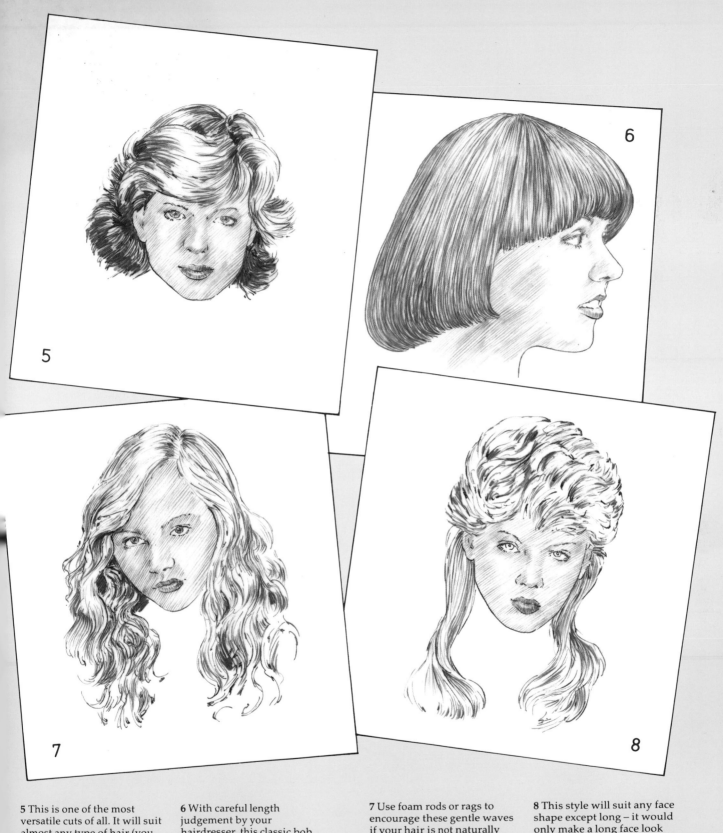

5 This is one of the most versatile cuts of all. It will suit almost any type of hair (you will need a body perm if your hair is very fine), and any face shape except a diamond shape. Blow-dry using a setting mousse if your hair needs extra body.

6 With careful length judgement by your hairdresser, this classic bob can suit any face shape except a square shape, as long as the hair is straight and not too coarse. An easy care style for daytime, it can quickly be changed for evenings using tongs or heated rollers.

7 Use foam rods or rags to encourage these gentle waves if your hair is not naturally wavy or end permed. This style is suitable for a round, oval, or diamond shape face, and any type of hair except coarse hair. Like all long hair, it requires you to take time and trouble to keep it looking its best.

8 This style will suit any face shape except long – it would only make a long face look longer. You need plenty of medium to coarse hair, and probably a body perm on the short, layered top section. Scrunch dry the top section using a setting mousse, and blow-dry the long bottom hair into smooth lines.

© DIAGRAM

Index